Sports Rehabilitation

Editor

JOE M. HART

CLINICS IN SPORTS MEDICINE

www.sportsmed.theclinics.com

Consulting Editor
MARK D. MILLER

April 2015 • Volume 34 • Number 2

ELSEVIER

1600 John F. Kennedy Boulevard • Suite 1800 • Philadelphia, Pennsylvania, 19103-2899

http://www.theclinics.com

CLINICS IN SPORTS MEDICINE Volume 34, Number 2
April 2015 ISSN 0278-5919, ISBN-13: 978-0-323-35985-6

Editor: Jennifer Flynn-Briggs
Developmental Editor: Donald Mumford

Clinics in Sports Medicine (ISSN 0278-5919) is published quarterly by Elsevier Inc., 360 Park Avenue South, New York, NY 10010-1710. Months of issue are January, April, July, and October. Business and Editorial Offices: 1600 John F. Kennedy Blvd., Ste. 1800, Philadelphia, PA 19103-2899. Customer Service Office: 3251 Riverport Lane, Maryland Heights, MO 63043. Periodicals postage paid at New York, NY and additional mailing offices. Subscription prices are $340.00 per year (US individuals), $540.00 per year (US institutions), $165.00 per year (US students), $385.00 per year (Canadian individuals), $666.00 per year (Canadian institutions), $235.00 (Canadian students), $470.00 per year (foreign individuals), $666.00 per year (foreign institutions), and $235.00 per year (foreign students). Foreign air speed delivery is included in all *Clinics* subscription prices. All prices are subject to change without notice. **POSTMASTER:** Send address changes to *Clinics in Sports Medicine*, Elsevier Health Sciences Division, Subscription Customer Service, 3251 Riverport Lane, Maryland Heights, MO 63043. Customer Service (orders, claims, online, change of address): Elsevier Health Sciences Division, Subscription Customer Service, 3251 Riverport Lane, Maryland Heights, MO 63043. Tel: 1-800-654-2452 (U.S. and Canada); 314-447-8871 (outside U.S. and Canada). Fax: 314-447-8029. E-mail: journalscustomerservice-usa@elsevier.com (for print support); journalsonlinesupport-usa@elsevier.com (for online support).

Reprints. For copies of 100 or more of articles in this publication, please contact the Commercial Reprints Department, Elsevier Inc., 360 Park Avenue South, New York, NY 10010-1710. Tel.: 212-633-3874; Fax: 212-633-3820; E-mail: reprints@elsevier.com.

Clinics in Sports Medicine is covered in *MEDLINE/PubMed (Index Medicus) Current Contents/Clinical Medicine, Excerpta Medica,* and *ISI/Biomed.*

Contributors

CONSULTING EDITOR

MARK D. MILLER, MD
S. Ward Casscells Professor, Head, Division of Sports Medicine, Department of Orthopaedic Surgery, University of Virginia; Team Physician, James Madison University, Charlottesville, Virginia

EDITOR

JOE M. HART, PhD, ATC
Associate Professor, Department of Kinesiology, Director of Clinical Research, Department of Orthopaedic Surgery, University of Virginia, Charlottesville, Virginia

AUTHORS

AMELIA J.H. ARUNDALE, PT, DPT, SCS
Biomechanics and Movement Science, University of Delaware, Newark, Delaware

ERICA BEIDLER, MEd, ATC
Department of Kinesiology, Michigan State University, East Lansing, Michigan

J. TROY BLACKBURN, PhD, ATC
Department of Exercise and Sport Science, University of North Carolina at Chapel Hill, Chapel Hill, North Carolina

STEVEN P. BROGLIO, PhD, ATC
School of Kinesiology, University of Michigan; University of Michigan Injury Center, Ann Arbor, Michigan

MICHAEL W. COLLINS, PhD
UPMC Sports Medicine Concussion Program, Department of Orthopaedic Surgery, University of Pittsburgh, Pittsburgh, Pennsylvania

TRACEY COVASSIN, PhD, ATC
Department of Kinesiology, Michigan State University, East Lansing, Michigan

CRAIG R. DENEGAR, PhD, PT, ATC, FNATA
Professor, Director, Doctor of Physical Therapy Program, Department of Kinesiology University of Connecticut, Storrs, Connecticut

MATHEW J. FAILLA, PT, MSPT, SCS
Biomechanics and Movement Science, University of Delaware, Newark, Delaware

MARK A. FEGER, MEd, ATC
Department of Kinesiology, University of Virginia, Charlottesville, Virginia

FRANÇOIS FOURCHET, PT, PhD
Senior Physiotherapist, Department of Physiotherapy, Hôpital La Tour Réseau de Soins, Geneva, Switzerland

JOHN J. FRASER, MS, PT, OCS
Department of Kinesiology, University of Virginia, Charlottesville, Virginia; US Navy Medicine Professional Development Center, Bethesda, Maryland

NEAL R. GLAVIANO, MEd, ATC
Departments of Kinesiology and Orthopaedic Surgery, University of Virginia, Charlottesville, Virginia

MATTHEW S. HARKEY, MS, ATC
Human Movement Sciences, University of North Carolina at Chapel Hill, Chapel Hill, North Carolina

JOE M. HART, PhD, ATC
Associate Professor, Department of Kinesiology, Director of Clinical Research, Department of Orthopaedic Surgery, University of Virginia, Charlottesville, Virginia

BRYAN C. HEIDERSCHEIT, PT, PhD
Professor, Department of Orthopedics and Rehabilitation; Department of Biomedical Engineering; Director of Research, Badger Athletic Performance; University of Wisconsin-Madison, Madison, Wisconsin

C. COLLIN HERB, MEd, ATC
Department of Kinesiology, University of Virginia, Charlottesville, Virginia

JAY HERTEL, PhD, ATC
Department of Kinesiology, University of Virginia, Charlottesville, Virginia

TODD R. HOOKS, PT, ATC, OCS, SCS, NREMT-1, CSCS, CMTPT, FAAOMPT
Champion Sports Medicine, A Physiotherapy Associates Clinic, Birmingham, Alabama

TYLER S. JOHNSTON, PT, DPT
Sports Medicine, University of Wisconsin Hospital and Clinics, Madison, Wisconsin

MICHAEL F. JOSEPH, PhD, PT
Assistant Professor, Doctor of Physical Therapy Program, Department of Kinesiology, University of Connecticut, Storrs, Connecticut

MICHAEL J. KISSENBERTH, MD
Vice Chair, Department of Orthopedics, Steadman-Hawkins Clinics of the Carolinas, Greenville Health System, Greenville, South Carolina

ANTHONY P. KONTOS, PhD
UPMC Sports Medicine Concussion Program, Department of Orthopaedic Surgery, University of Pittsburgh, Pittsburgh, Pennsylvania

JIACHENG LI, BS
Department of Orthopaedic Surgery, University of Virginia, Charlottesville, Virginia

DAVID S. LOGERSTEDT, PT, PhD, SCS
Biomechanics and Movement Science Program, University of Delaware, Delaware; Assistant Professor, Department of Physical Therapy, University of the Sciences in Philadelphia, Philadelphia, Pennsylvania

BRITTNEY A. LUC, MS, ATC
Human Movement Sciences, University of North Carolina at Chapel Hill, Chapel Hill, North Carolina

PATRICK O. McKEON, PhD, ATC, CSCS
Assistant Professor, Department of Exercise and Sport Sciences, Ithaca College, Ithaca, New York

ANNE MUCHA, DPT
UPMC Sports Medicine Concussion Program, Department of Orthopaedic Surgery, University of Pittsburgh; UPMC Centers for Rehab Services, UPMC, Pittsburgh, Pennsylvania

JENNIFER OSTROWSKI, PhD, ATC
Department of Health, Promotion, and Human Performance, Weber State University, Ogden, Utah

DEREK N. PAMUKOFF, MS
Human Movement Sciences, University of North Carolina at Chapel Hill, Chapel Hill, North Carolina

BRIAN PIETROSIMONE, PhD, ATC
Department of Exercise and Sport Science, University of North Carolina at Chapel Hill, Chapel Hill, North Carolina

MARCUS A. ROTHERMICH, MD
Department of Orthopaedic Surgery, Washington University, St Louis, Missouri

MICHAEL A. SHAFFER, MSPT, OCS, ATC
Coordinator of Sports Rehabilitation, University of Iowa Sports Medicine, Clinical Specialist, Department of Rehabilitation Therapies, University of Iowa Hospitals and Clinics, Iowa City, Iowa

MARC A. SHERRY, PT, DPT, LAT
Sports Medicine, University of Wisconsin Hospital and Clinics, Madison, Wisconsin

LYNN SNYDER-MACKLER, PT, ScD, SCS, FAPTA
Biomechanics and Movement Science; Department of Physical Therapy, University of Delaware, Newark, Delaware

CHARLES A. THIGPEN, PT, PhD, ATC
Clinical Research Scientist, Proaxis Therapy; Director of Observational Clinical Research in Orthopedics, Center for Rehabilitation and Reconstruction Sciences, Greenville, South Carolina

JESSICA WALLACE, MA, ATC
Department of Kinesiology, Michigan State University, East Lansing, Michigan

KEVIN E. WILK, PT, DPT, FAPTA
Champion Sports Medicine, A Physiotherapy Associates Clinic, Birmingham, Alabama; Rehabilitation Consultant, Tampa Bay Rays Baseball Team, Tampa Bay, Florida; Director of Rehabilitative Research, American Sports Medicine Institute, Birmingham, Alabama

RICHELLE M. WILLIAMS, MS, ATC
School of Kinesiology, University of Michigan, Ann Arbor, Michigan

Contents

When an athlete is injured, the primary focus of the sports medicine team is to treat the physical effects of the injury. However, many injured athletes experience negative psychological responses that should also be addressed throughout the rehabilitation process. Sports medicine professions should use psychosocial skills to help decrease the negative consequences of the injury, such as fear of reinjury, anxiety, depression, and adherence to rehabilitation. These psychosocial skills include goal setting, imagery, relaxation techniques, motivation, and self-talk. This article addresses the negative consequences of injury, psychosocial skills used to aid in the rehabilitation process, and clinical implications of the psychological aspects of rehabilitation in sport.

Concussion is one of the most hotly debated topics in sports medicine today. Research surrounding concussion has experienced significant growth recently, especially in the areas of incidence, assessment, and recovery. However, there is limited research on the most effective rehabilitation approaches for this injury. This review evaluates the current literature for evidence for and against physical and cognitive rest and the emerging areas targeting vestibular, oculomotor, and pharmacologic interventions for the rehabilitation of sport-related concussion.

Rotator cuff repairs have increased. Although clinical trials have examined the effect of immobilization and timing of passive range of motion (ROM) on patient outcomes and structural integrity, there is controversy as to the timing and progression for therapy. Primary goals are restoring function while maintaining the structural integrity of the repair. We advocate for a protocol of 4 to 6 weeks of immobilization, followed by protected passive ROM, which is followed by a gradual progression to active ROM and then appropriate resistance exercise program for most all rotator cuff repairs. The rate of progression should be adjusted individually.

often involve a comprehensive evaluation that includes assessing the chronicity of the pain, the specific location of the complaint, and the previous treatment modalities attempted by the patient. This common diagnosis includes a wide variety of different pathologic abnormalities that can be present independently or concomitantly and cause a spectrum of disabilities for the patient.

In competitive sports medicine, supervised rehabilitation is the standard of care; in the general population, unsupervised home exercise is more common. We systematically reviewed randomized, controlled trials comparing outcomes for supervised rehabilitation versus home exercise programs. Supervised rehabilitation programs resulted in (1) less pain and subjective instability, (2) greater gains in ankle strength and joint position sense, and (3) inconclusive results regarding prevention of recurrent ankle sprains. We recommend supervised rehabilitation over home exercise programs owing to the improved short-term patient-recorded evidence with a strength-of-recommendation taxonomy level of evidence of 2B.

The intrinsic muscles of the foot play a critical role in the regulation of absorption and propulsion during dynamic activities. Dysfunction of these may lead to an increased demand on the remaining components within the foot core system to maintain dynamic foot control, leading to a more rapid breakdown of these contributors and those proximal to the foot. Training the intrinsic foot muscles through a systematic progression of isolation via the short foot exercise offers the opportunity to reincorporate their contribution into the foot core system. This article discusses the function of the intrinsic foot muscles, their contributions to dynamic foot control, and a progressive training paradigm.

Tendinopathy is a common and complex disorder. Once viewed as an inflammatory condition labeled tendinitis, it is now viewed along a continuum that can lead to tissue necrosis and risk of tendon rupture. Anti-inflammatory medications can alter symptoms but may also promote tissue degeneration. Loading of the tendon through exercise, especially exercise involving eccentric muscle contraction, has been shown to promote symptom resolution and functional recovery in many patients. This article reviews the pathoetiology of tendinopathy and the role anti-inflammatory interventions and therapeutic exercise in treatment of active patients.

Sports Rehabilitation

CLINICS IN SPORTS MEDICINE

Foreword

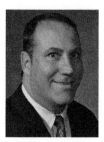

Mark D. Miller, MD
Consulting Editor

This issue literally comes from my Hart...Joe Hart, that is, Dr Hart and his wife, Jen Hart (PA-C), have been affiliated with our Sports Medicine Division at the University of Virginia for over a decade. The numerous contributions that both have made to patient care/education/satisfaction and to musculoskeletal provider education are significant. This current issue of *Clinics in Sports Medicine* is certainly no exception. Dr Hart has invited a veritable Who's Who in musculoskeletal rehabilitation to bring us up to speed in this rapidly evolving science. As he notes in his *Preface*, this treatise covers the gambit of rehabilitation—literally from Head to Toe! To all clinicians out there, a special footnote—good results are directly correlated with good rehab! Thank-you to Dr Hart and all authors who have contributed to this issue!

Mark D. Miller, MD
Division of Sports Medicine
Department of Orthopaedic Surgery
University of Virginia
400 Ray C. Hunt Dr, Suite 330
Charlottesville, VA 22908-0159, USA

James Madison University
Harrisonburg, VA 22807, USA

E-mail address:
MDM3P@hscmail.mcc.virginia.edu

Clin Sports Med 34 (2015) xi
http://dx.doi.org/10.1016/j.csm.2015.02.002
0278-5919/15/$ – see front matter © 2015 Published by Elsevier Inc.

Preface

Sports Rehabilitation

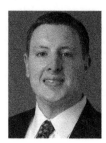

Joe M. Hart, PhD, ATC
Editor

This issue of *Clinics in Sports Medicine* highlights many current concepts and controversies in sports medicine and orthopedic rehabilitation. Rehabilitation is central to optimizing outcomes following both acute and chronic injury, especially in those who lead active lifestyles whether due to desire to stay healthy, sports involvement, or work. When injuries occur, our patients often seek treatment with the goal of returning to preinjury level or type of activity as quickly as possible. Rehabilitation specialists seek evidence-based approaches to manage patients through recovery and toward individual patient goals. Wherever your particular position in the realm of sports medicine, we all strive to bring the best and most current therapies to provide the best outcomes for our patients. As scholars and clinicians, we are also responsible for testing hypotheses, critiquing results, and sharing viewpoints through dissemination and debate.

In this issue, we recruited well-known and respected clinicians and scientists who are each leaders in their respective fields. Each has provided a current view of research and clinical practice related to their respective areas of expertise and experience. Each of these articles is informative and applicable to clinical practice and scholarship that will inspire discussion and debate. The issue spans from head to foot, literally. Articles ranging from sports psychology, tendinopathy, concussion, shoulder, thigh, knee, and ankle—any sports medicine professional will benefit from each of these thorough and

Clin Sports Med 34 (2015) xiii–xiv
http://dx.doi.org/10.1016/j.csm.2015.02.001
0278-5919/15/$ – see front matter © 2015 Published by Elsevier Inc.

sportsmed.theclinics.com

insightful reviews. So, without further delay, I invite you to enjoy this issue of *Clinics in Sports Medicine*, learn from the experts, and engage in a professional debate with your peers.

Joe M. Hart, PhD, ATC
Department of Kinesiology
Department of Orthopaedic Surgery
University of Virginia
Charlottesville, VA, USA

E-mail address:
joehart@virginia.edu

Psychosocial Aspects of Rehabilitation in Sports

Tracey Covassin, PhD, ATC[a],*, Erica Beidler, MEd, ATC[a],
Jennifer Ostrowski, PhD, ATC[b], Jessica Wallace, MA, ATC[a]

KEYWORDS

• Psychosocial skills • Rehabilitation • Injury • Psychological recovery

KEY POINTS

- Awareness of the psychosocial response to athletic injury helps clinicians to effectively assist patients with the healing and recovery process.
- Patients with high trait anxiety tend to have high state anxiety and this may influence thoughts and feelings about the injury and healing process.
- Fear of reinjury can have a negative influence on the rehabilitation process because of concerns about returning to preinjury level, especially as the patient gets closer to return-to-play.
- Effective communication skills in the athletic training setting are a key component to patient care.
- Clinicians must focus on the injured person, rather than the physical injury. There are several psychosocial techniques to choose from to ensure a holistic treatment of each individual.

INTRODUCTION: NATURE OF THE PROBLEM

Injury is an inherent consequence of athletic participation. Athletic injury not only affects patients' physical well-being, but also their self-concept, self-esteem, belief system, values, commitments, and emotional equilibrium.[1] Often, sports medicine professionals focus on the physical damage from injury, while ignoring the psychosocial aspects of injury and the thoughts, feelings, and behaviors associated with an injury.[2] Athletic injury can be an imposing source of stress, and patients often experience feelings of tension, confusion, hostility, loneliness, fear, irritability, and anxiety.[3] Furthermore, feelings of guilt and being ignored often accompany athletic injury because patients feel isolated and estranged from their team and their sport.[4] Research has demonstrated a positive relationship between injury severity and

[a] Department of Kinesiology, Michigan State University, 308 West Circle Drive, East Lansing, MI 48824, USA; [b] Department of Health, Promotion, and Human Performance, Weber State University, 302 E Swenson Building, Ogden, UT 84408, USA
* Corresponding author.
E-mail address: covassin@msu.edu

Clin Sports Med 34 (2015) 199–212
http://dx.doi.org/10.1016/j.csm.2014.12.004
0278-5919/15/$ – see front matter © 2015 Elsevier Inc. All rights reserved.
sportsmed.theclinics.com

negative mood in patients.[5] As a result, several theoretic models have emerged that suggest that cognitive and affective factors may contribute to rehabilitation outcomes.[6] Therefore, an understanding of how patients respond to injury and rehabilitation assists clinicians when treating injured patients.[7]

The integrated model of psychological response to the sport injury and rehabilitation process[8] is a conceptual model of injury response to an interrelated psychosocial process of cognition, affect, and behavior **Fig. 1**.[9] According to this model, injury

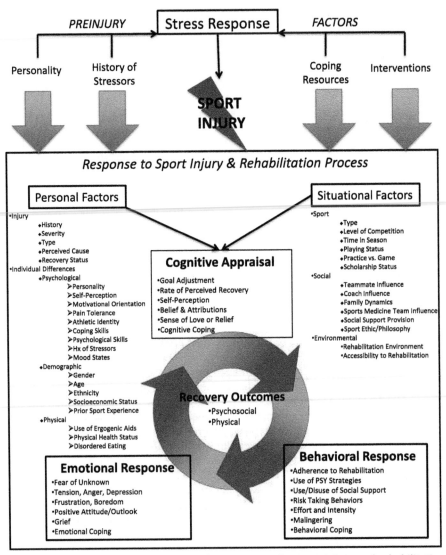

Fig. 1. Integrated model of psychological response to the sport injury and rehabilitation process. HX, history; PSY, psychology. (*From* Wiese-Bjornstal D, Smith A, Shaffer S, et al. An integrated model of response to sport injury: psychological and sociological dynamics. J Appl Sport Psychol 1998;10(1):49; with permission.)

becomes a new stressor in the patient's life, leading to thoughts, feelings, and actions that affect rehabilitation outcomes.[9] Also affecting the injury response are a variety of interacting personal and individual differences, such as age, sex, injury history, characteristics of personality, and interactions with medical professionals.[9] Cognitive appraisal postinjury involves the many assessments patients make regarding their sense of self, identity, loss, optimism, challenge, or burnout. These appraisals influence a patient's affect-related psychosocial responses of emotion and behavior, and physical recovery.[9] Emotional or affective responses to injury often include mood disturbances, such as depression, anxiety, low vigor, fatigue, grief, burnout, and ultimately fear of reinjury.[9]

Cognition and emotions influence behavior during the rehabilitation process, such as attendance at rehabilitation sessions, rehabilitation adherence, substance abuse, exercise dependence, and even suicidal behavior.[9] There is a significant amount of evidence that suggests that a patient's motivation to take on rehabilitation of an injury is a critical factor that determines treatment adherence.[10] Awareness of the psychosocial response to athletic injury helps clinicians empathize and assist patients to cope effectively and prevent adverse responses to injury that may disrupt the healing and recovery process.[7] Proper rehabilitation that includes the psychosocial components and an understanding of factors that may contribute to a patient's response to injury is essential to facilitate a holistic recovery and prevent further injury.

NEGATIVE CONSEQUENCES OF INJURY
Anxiety

Anxiety is a common psychosocial response to injury.[11] Trait anxiety refers to how a person feels in general toward various situations that may influence anxiety levels.[12] State anxiety describes how a person feels in the current moment about various situations that may influence anxiety levels.[12] Patients who have high trait anxiety tend to have high state anxiety postinjury.[13] Leddy and coworkers[13] examined the psychosocial impact of injury in male Division I university athletes. Injured athletes reported higher levels of anxiety compared with noninjured patients at immediate postinjury assessment and at 2 months. Injured patients may exhibit anxiety related to pain, before surgery, and when returning to competition.[14,15] Such factors as injury severity and time loss from practice or competition can influence whether or not patients experience high or low levels of state anxiety.[3] Moreover, injured patients experience anxiety as a result of loss of social support from teammates or coaches, or anxiety may be associated with the perception of letting down family members, friends, coaches, and teammates.[15] Health care professionals can alleviate anxiety by using psychosocial techniques, such as relaxation, imagery, goal setting, and positive self-talk.

Stress

Injury is generally perceived as a negative life event, and as such it becomes a major source of stress for patients. Stress is defined as the demands of a situation exceeding the resources to respond to those demands.[12] For example, a patient who sustains an injury and cannot deal with the issues surrounding this situation is likely to experience stress. Physiologically, stress causes narrowing of attention, increased distractibility, and higher levels of muscle tension,[16] all of which can have a negative impact on healing and rehabilitation. Stressors come in three different forms: (1) physical, (2) social, and (3) performance.[14,17] Physical stressors include such issues as regaining overall fitness level and having to make technical adjustments to accommodate the injury (eg, how to get around campus using crutches).[17,18] If the injured patient is removed from participation, he or she may also experience social stressors, such as being isolated from team activities, feeling pressure to return to play from their support system (eg, teammates, coaches, parents, friends), attempting to uphold their athletic reputation, or being passed by lesser skilled players. From a performance standpoint, injury can lead to fear of falling behind their teammates or beliefs that they may not be able reach their preinjury level of athletic performance.[17,19,20] Performance stressors are even more amplified in elite athletic settings where the patient is unsure if their injury will cause them to be cut from their team, which could directly affect their monetary stability and future career opportunities.[17,20] The relationship of perceived stress and injury, in addition to the stress response that patients may have following injury, carry many important implications. When considering the health and wellness of patients, it is important to understand the cause and effect relationship between perceived stress and injury, and the negative impacts of stress on recovery and rehabilitation processes. Patients can be taught techniques to properly manage their stress, including goal setting, self-talk, imagery, and relaxation techniques.

Depression

Research has suggested that more than 20% of Division I collegiate athletes experience general symptoms of depression.[21] Those with moderate to severe injury reported emotional fluctuations, anxiety, anger, and frustration.[2] Specifically, injured athletes have exhibited higher depression symptoms than noninjured athletes up to 2 months following injury.[13] Some of these injured athletes reported psychosocial issues that would warrant referral to a mental health professional.[13]

Several researchers have suggest that increased incidence of depression has been associated with a history of concussion in retired boxers[22] and professional football players.[23] Moreover, elevated levels of depression and mood disturbances have been documented in concussed patients.[24,25] Mainwaring and colleagues[25] found that concussed patients reported three times greater total mood disturbance and depression compared with their baseline depression scores. Furthermore, collegiate and high school concussed patients demonstrated depression symptoms 14 days postinjury. It is extremely important for health care professionals to be cognizant of depression issues related to injury and know when to refer to a clinical psychologist for further assistance.

Adherence to Rehabilitation

Injury rehabilitation can be a long process, and it can be difficult to keep athletes motivated and adherent for the duration of the treatment. Some ways to increase rehabilitation adherence are to use effective communication skills to educate the patient on their injury and care plan, engage patients in relaxation exercises to decrease the stress and anxiety related to their injury, use a collaborative goal-setting process that takes individual needs into account, and introduce performance imagery to help visualize what it will be like when they return to play.[26]

Some injured patients may have weak, inappropriate, or no motivation to get better, such as a third-string player who does not get to compete in games. These individuals may actually be motivated to malinger (ie, not want to get better or return to competition) and not adhere to their rehabilitation plan because they are receiving more attention for being injured compared with when they are not injured. This is a difficult situation for health care professionals to deal with because there is no physical reason for their reported symptoms. Athletic trainers may have the most experience dealing with this phenomenon because they work closely with their patients on a daily basis and are constantly monitoring for signs and symptoms of decline during the injury recovery process. Returning to the previous scenario where the individual is receiving attention for being injured, it can be helpful to only acknowledge and praise positive expressions and actions that move them toward recovery. It may also be useful to get the coach and team involved in this situation. If they can make the patient feel like they have an important accessory role to the team, then their motives to get better may change in a positive way.

Fear of Reinjury

Fear of reinjury can have a negative influence on the rehabilitation process because of concerns about returning to preinjury sport level.[27] Specifically, as patients get closer to returning to sport participation, their fear of reinjury increases.[18,19,28–31] Moreover, fear of reinjury can lead to lower sport confidence, failure to "give 100%" during rehabilitation or sport, or fear of being placed in an injury-provoking situation.[32] Fear of reinjury has also been a reason for athletes stopping or retiring from their sport.[14,17,28,33–35] Specifically, McCullough and colleagues[34] reported that 52% of high school athletes and 50% of collegiate athletes who had anterior cruciate ligament (ACL) reconstructive surgery did not return to sport participation because of fear of reinjury. It is important for health care professionals to recognize patients who demonstrate a fear of reinjury, because this could potentially lead to lack of self-confidence, further injury (eg, recall the relationship between stress and injury), or cessation of sport participation. Effective communication, self-talk (including reframing), imagery, and relaxation are some psychosocial skills that may decrease the patient's fear of reinjury.

PSYCHOSOCIAL INTERVENTION TECHNIQUES
Effective Communication

Because of the stressful and time-sensitive nature of athletic injuries, it can be difficult for health care professionals to educate and coordinate the plan of care with all the involved personal (eg, patient, physicians, and parents). However, effective communication between patients, health care professionals, and physicians is a key component for patient-oriented collaborative care.[36] A review of 16 studies on communication in the medical field concluded that having effective physician-patient communication correlates to improved health outcomes for patients.[37]

To improve on effective communication skills in the athletic training setting, clinicians may seek guidance from the "4Es" of the Bayer educational model (engage, empathize, educate, enlist) in addition to the basic "2Fs" of biomedical tasks (find the problem, fix the problem) (**Fig. 2**).[38] To develop an open line of communication, the clinician must first *engage* the recipients (patients, coaches, health care professionals, and so forth) in a language that is familiar and relatable to them. During this time, it is important to build personal connections and focus on the individual as a person, not as an injury. The next communication task is to *empathize* with the individual and understand their viewpoints on the situation. Actively listen to the values and concerns of the involved parties while being "present" and "with" them at all times. Be aware of your body language (eg, eye contact, gestures of understanding) and make an attempt to minimize distractions (eg, do not write when they are talking, put your cell phone away, talk in a quiet place away from the treatment area).

Once a connection has been made and the individual's needs are known, *education* on the details of the injury should follow, the individual should be given the opportunity to ask questions, and the health care professional should check for their understanding of important information. When educating about an injury it is important to

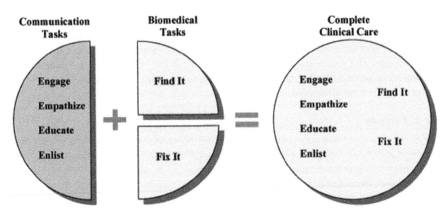

Fig. 2. "4Es" of the Bayer educational model. (*From* Keller VF, Carroll JG. A new model for physician-patient communication. Patient Educ Couns 1994;23:131–40; with permission.)

remember that each person has a previous knowledge set about the situation, so finding out what they already know and believe can be helpful when designing the comprehensive plan of care. There is a large amount of information that must be communicated following injury, but the individual will have a limited capacity of information that they can internalize in a single session. Education should be broken into manageable doses, and the order of information delivered should be prioritized (ie, most important information delivered first and possibly repeatedly).

The last communication component is to *enlist* the patient and health care team members in the decision-making process and construction of an adherence strategy for rehabilitation. Rather than telling each person what their role is and what needs to be done, allow them to express their thoughts and feeling on how they feel they can contribute to the injury plan of care. With your guidance, allow the patient to come up with a rehabilitation regimen (including engaging the patient in the goal-setting process) that they think will work for them. Enlisting them to get involved and give their feedback could provide the patient with an internal sense of control over the injury process and it is hoped make them more likely to adhere to the plan they have helped create.

Goal Setting

Setting goals is an innate process that is used in all aspects of life, and one that is easily transferable to the rehabilitation setting. Patients and rehabilitation professionals have endorsed goal setting as an effective means of enhancing motivation.[39,40] Although we set goals frequently, it is important to recognize that this is a psychosocial skill that can be strengthened through education and practice. The goal setting skills that patients have learned to improve their sport performance may be easily translated and incorporated into the injury recovery process. The primary negative psychosocial responses of injured patients include stress and anxiety, anger, and treatment adherence problems.[11,13,41] A recent study of athletic trainers found that goal setting was perceived to be among the top two psychosocial strategies in addressing these issues.[41] In fact, according to the literature, goal setting is the strategy that is most often endorsed by sport psychology and sports medicine professionals[42] and is one of the most commonly used psychosocial strategies during injury rehabilitation.[43] Goal setting has been shown to have a positive effect on increasing patient motivation and rehabilitation adherence and compliance.[44]

To use goal setting effectively for rehabilitation, it is first important to recognize that there are three main types of goals to consider: (1) outcome goals, (2) performance goals, and (3) process goals.[45,46] Outcome goals are those that focus on the outcome of the event, such as successfully returning to athletic participation following an ACL reconstruction.[12] Performance goals concentrate on short-term performance objectives that must be met to achieve the overall outcome goal.[12] In ACL rehabilitation, a performance goal may be to increase knee flexion range of motion by 10 degrees compared with the previous measurement the week before. Lastly, process goals deal with the individual components that need to be present to perform a skill well.[12] For the ACL example, a process goal would be to regain quadriceps function in the early stages of postoperative rehabilitation by consciously contracting the quadriceps during quad sets and straight leg raises.

Not only do all three goal types need to be considered when defining the short- and long-term goals of the injury care plan, but care must be taken in how the goals are formulated and set. The importance of getting the patient involved in the goal setting process should not be overlooked. By using effective communication techniques to educate the injured patient about the recovery process, goal setting becomes a team effort that allows the patient's thoughts, feelings, and ideas to be taken into consideration. The following are basic principles that can increase the effectiveness of goal setting in the rehabilitation setting[12]:

- Set specific goals
- Set moderately difficult but realistic goals
- Set long- and short-term goals
- Set performance, process, and outcome goals
- Write goals down
- Develop specific plans to achieve goals
- Consider the patient's personality and motivation
- Foster an individual's goal commitment
- Provide goal support
- Provide evaluation of and feedback about goals

Goal setting is also commonly considered a form of social support that can be provided by health care professionals. Research suggests that social support in the form of emotional and task support (including goal setting) were most helpful to injured patients during the early phases of rehabilitation when pain and swelling were less predictable. Additionally, performance and process goals were used to aid in the loss of athletic identity. As rehabilitation progressed, goal setting was used to facilitate rehabilitation adherence.[29]

Self-Talk

Self-talk is anything that an individual says out loud or thinks (nonverbally) about themselves.[47] Self-talk occurs in three forms: (1) positive, (2) negative, and (3) instructional. Positive self-talk (eg, "I can do this!") is used in sport to focus or refocus the attention, to increase motivation, and to promote an overall positive attitude during play. Conversely, negative self-talk (eg, "I stink at this!") should be avoided because it is detrimental to performance, fosters anxiety, and promotes self-doubt. The third type of self-talk is different from the other types because it does not directly affect motivation. The purpose of instructional self-talk (eg, "Keep your eye on the ball!") is to focus on and break down technical or task-related aspects of sport to increase performance.[12] Health care professionals working with injured athletes should work to minimize negative self-talk and increase positive and instructional self-talk to break bad habits, initiate action, sustain effort, and acquire new skills in the physically active population.[12]

Promoting positive self-talk techniques throughout rehabilitation is a simple way for clinicians to actively combat negative self-talk. First, the individual must identify when they are engaging in negative self-talk. Ask your patient to write down any negative comments that they may have thought or said during the day, or specifically during a session of rehabilitation. This exercise helps them to become aware of their negative self-talk tendencies and the situations that may trigger this response. From there, the concept of thought stopping should be used. Instruct the patient to come up with a simple trigger word or phrase to be used immediately after they have a negative thought, such as "Stop!" Next the patient should develop a trigger word that will be used to interrupt the negative thought. Once the negative thought is identified and stopped, the final phase is to replace it with positive self-talk. One strategy for this is to have your patient refer back to their negative self-talk list and come up with a simple positive replacement phase. Replacement phases should be realistically positive to be viewed as a meaningful replacement.[12,48]

Imagery

For decades, research has shown a positive effect of psychosocial skills on the rehabilitation process. One of the most iconic studies to demonstrate an effect on healing was conducted by Ievleva and Orlick[44] in 1991. This study found that fast-healing patients (those who healed from knee and ankle injuries in fewer than 5 weeks) were more likely to have used psychosocial skills, such as goal setting, positive self-talk, and healing imagery, compared with slow-healing patients (those whose injuries required more than 16 weeks to heal).[44] Several researchers have suggested that using imagery results in a faster recovery time from injury.[49,50] Moreover, imagery has been shown to positively relate to self-efficacy[51] and results in decreased patient anxiety.[52]

Imagery is traditionally a mental preparation technique used to create or recreate experiences within the mind to increase performance. Imagery is also commonly referred to as visualization, mental rehearsal, simulation, and mental training.[12] In general, patients use imagery for motivational (ie, goal-oriented responses, arousal control) and cognitive (ie, skill practice, strategy formation) benefits during sport participation.[53] Some specific reasons for using imagery are to improve concentration, build confidence, enhance motivation, control emotional responses, acquire and practice sport skills, acquire and practice performance strategy, cope with pain and injury, and solve problems.[12,54] These same uses are applicable during the injury recovery process. In addition to helping patients overcome physical pain, imagery may be an effective way to improve the overall affect and outlook of patients.

As a clinician, it is important to educate injured patients that imagery is a skill that can be improved on with practice.[55] It does not come naturally to everyone, so patients should be reassured not to be discouraged if this technique is challenging at first. The primary components of effective imagery are vividness and controllability. To create vivid and realistic images, as many senses as possible (ie, sight, sound, smell, touch, taste, body positioning) should be included to paint a detailed image of the experience and environment.[12] This also includes attaching appropriate emotional responses and moods to the mental rehearsal.[12] To learn more about imagery and how to apply it in clinical practice see the *Routledge Handbook of Applied Sport Psychology*[47] and the *Psychological Bases of Sport Injuries* textbooks.[56]

Pain management, healing, and return to play imagery are specific visualization skills that can be incorporated into injury rehabilitation. When determining what types of imagery to use, a health care professional should first determine the nature of the task, skill level of the patient, and the patient's ability to imagine.[12,57] Different situations call for different types of imagery, because the goals of an imagery script are different for individuals in the acute phase of injury (ie, internal tissue healing visualization) compared with someone who is nearing return to play (ie, sport-specific tasks). There are different uses of imagery for injury prevention, immediately postinjury, and during rehabilitation. A patient who has had previous training in imagery likely has a higher ability to imagine compared with patients who have not.[57] Some quick ways to objectively gauge the imagery skill level of patients are to use the Sport Imagery Questionnaire and the Sport Imagery Ability Measure.[58,59] It may also be helpful to pair mental rehearsal with physical skills to enhance overall effectiveness.[60] For example, instruct the patient to visualize their individual muscle fibers contracting and shortening as they move the weight upward during bicep curls. No rehabilitation process is complete without frequent reevaluations of progress and adjustments to task difficulty, and imagery is no different. Changing up imagery scripts to satisfy the evolving individual needs, abilities, and interests of the patient keeps them interested and challenges them to improve not only physically, but also mentally.

Relaxation Techniques

Stressful situations cause narrowing of attention, increased distractibility, and higher levels of muscle tension,[16] all of which have negative impacts on the rehabilitation process. The use of deep breathing or voluntary muscle relaxation techniques during physical rehabilitation has been shown to decrease anxiety and pain, and to speed physical recovery.[49] The addition of stress inoculation training (ie, a cognitive-behavioral intervention including deep breathing, muscle relaxation, imagery, and positive self-talk) to a physical rehabilitation program produced significant differences in state anxiety and pain in the patient group. The average number of days to recovery (criterion, 80% of uninvolved knee strength) was also significantly less in the intervention group.[49] More recently, the use of physical (deep breathing) or cognitive (mental imagery) relaxation techniques have been shown to be equally effective at decreasing perceived (ie, 1–10 Likert scale) and physiologic (ie, cortisol level in saliva) levels of stress compared with a control group that listened only to nature sounds (ie, ocean with occasional seagulls calling).[61]

Patients who continue to focus on the physical, social, and performance stressors associated with injury may not be able to fully relax, clear their minds, and focus their attention on the rehabilitation tasks that they are performing. To combat these stressors, clinicians can introduce relaxation techniques (ie, breathing control, progressive muscle relaxation, and meditation) early in the injury care plan and carry them through the process until full return to participation is achieved. The key to relaxation is the use of proper breathing techniques.[12] These techniques can be taught quickly and used any time during the rehabilitation routine for a short mental break to regain composure and control. Breath control training should focus on smooth, deep, and rhythmic breathing with diaphragm movement and slow exhalation. To teach this skill, instruct patients to divide their lungs into three parts: (1) lower, (2) middle, and (3) upper. First have them focus on filling the lower portion of their lungs by pushing their abdomen out and lowering their diaphragm. To fill the middle third, train them to expand their chest cavity outward and slightly raise their rib cage. To finish the inhalation phase have them continue to breath inward until their chest and shoulders raise and no more air can enter. Prompt them to hold the inhalation phase for a few seconds before slowly exhaling by lowering the ribs and shoulders, sucking in their abdomen, and allowing their diaphragm to rise back to its resting position. The inhalation and exhalation process should occur at 1:2 ratio to slow breathing and increase the patient's relaxation and focus.[62] Another type of stress-reducing technique to incorporate into clinical athletic training is progressive muscle relaxation. Jacobson[63] provides a detailed script of progressive relaxation exercises that can be adapted for use in the athletic training room.

Motivation

Motivation is defined as the direction and intensity of one's efforts toward something,[64] where direction refers to the attraction to situations and intensity of effort refers to how much energy is concentrated to a specific situation. An example of high motivation is an injured patient who is always on time for their rehabilitation session and completes each task to the absolute best of their ability. As health care professionals, we appreciate our highly motivated patients because it makes our job and the rehabilitation process easier. The real challenge is how to manage unmotivated patients who often miss rehabilitation sessions and, when they do attend, tend to just go through the motions of their exercises. The use of effective communication skills, goal setting, imagery, and self-talk are all ways to motivate patients throughout injury care. By making the patient an active part of the process, rather than just instructing them what to do on a daily basis, the patient is given a sense of ownership and investment in the goals and plan that they have set for themselves.

Motivation can change from day to day and there are many individual differences to consider. Some ways that health care professionals can increase the motivation of their patients is to provide experiences that ensure success, give rewards based on performance effort, use verbal and nonverbal appraisals, change up the content and order of exercises, involve the patient in the decision-making process, and help them set realistic goals.[12] When developing a rehabilitation program, health care professionals must keep the individual's personality and current surroundings in mind. For example, some injured patients may need a large support group around them to get motivated, whereas others are more motivated when they are on their own. Health care professionals can also change the environment to enhance motivation of the injured patient. For example, you could pair two similarly injured patients up to work on their rehabilitation together (ie, peer modeling) or you could use goal-setting to generate competition versus their own previous performances.

CLINICAL APPLICATION OF PSYCHOSOCIAL TECHNIQUES

When attempting to develop and implement a psychosocial skills program, health care professionals should consider that techniques may be used as stand-alone interventions, or may be combined based on the patient's needs. Consider the use of therapeutic modalities when a patient is injured. To decrease pain, accomplish rehabilitation goals, and aid recovery, one may use several modalities at once, or one may focus on just one. With modalities, we may choose one over another because we believe it will work better with a particular patient, or because we have had success with it in the past. The same decision-making process should be implemented when using psychosocial skills. In a given situation with a given patient, several techniques may be equally effective at reaching a goal. One may choose to use several techniques, or may find that a certain skill works better with a particular patient. Regardless of the technique that is used, maintaining a focus on the psychosocial aspects of injury facilitates greater holistic treatment of the patient.

SUMMARY

There are many psychosocial factors that influence healing and the success of rehabilitation, including a patient's self-confidence and self-efficacy; perceptions of control over the process; a patient's motivation and effort with the prescribed rehabilitation program; perception of pain; and patient anxiety, fear, and worry. It is the goal of psychosocial skills to provide the patient with a greater perception of control over the healing and rehabilitation processes, and to provide them with skills that can facilitate physical rehabilitation, and skills that can alter their perception of pain. To best equip the injured patient with the appropriate coping skills, the clinician must first understand how each individual patient responds to injury and then provide skills that meet individual needs. Communication must remain constant to effectively meet individual needs of each injured patient, and this will allow for a holistic approach to rehabilitation.

REFERENCES

1. Danish S. Psychological aspects in the care and treatment of athletic injuries. Littleton (MA): PSG Publishing Company; 1986.
2. Tracey J. The emotional responses to the injury and rehabilitation process. J Appl Sport Psychol 2003;15:279–93.
3. Udry E, Gould D, Bridges D, et al. Down but not out: athlete responses to season-ending injuries. J Sport Exerc Psychol 1997;19(3):229–48.
4. Mainwaring L. Restoration of self: a model for the psychological response of athletes to severe knee injuries. Can J Rehabil 1999;12(3):145–54.
5. Smith A, Scott S, O'Fallon W, et al. Emotional responses of athletes to injury. Mayo Clin Proc 1990;65(1):38–50.
6. Tripp D, Stanish W, Ebel-Lam A, et al. Fear of reinjury, negative affect, and catastrophizing predicting return to sport in recreational athletes with anterior cruciate ligament injuries at 1 year postsurgery. Rehabil Psychol 2007;52(1):74–81.
7. Walker N, Thatcher J, Lavallee D. Psychological responses to injury in competitive sport: a critical review. J R Soc Health 2007;127(4):174–80.
8. Wiese-Bjornstal D, Smith A, Shaffer S, et al. An integrated model of response to sport injury: psychological and sociological dynamics. J Appl Sport Psychol 1998;10(1):46–69.
9. Wiese-Bjornstal D. Psychology and socioculture affect injury risk, response, and recovery in high-intensity athletes: a consensus statement. Scand J Med Sci Sports 2010;20(2):103–11.
10. Hagger M, Chatzisarantis N, Griffin M. Injury representations, coping, emotions, and functional outcomes in athletes with sports-related injuries: a test of self-regulation theory. J Appl Soc Psychol 2005;35(11):2345–74.
11. Larson G, Starkey C, Zaichkowsky L. Psychological aspects of athletic injuries as perceived by athletic trainers. Sport Psychol 1996;10:15–24.
12. Weinberg R, Gould D, editors. Foundations in sport and exercise psychology. Champaign (IL): Human Kinetics; 2011.
13. Leddy M, Lambert M, Ogles B. Psychological consequences of athletic injury among high-level competitors. Res Q Exerc Sport 1994;65:347–54.
14. Podlog L, Dimmock J, Miller J. A review of return to sport concerns following injury rehabilitation: practitioner strategies for enhancing recovery outcomes. Phys Ther Sport 2011;12:36–42.
15. Cassidy C. Understanding sport-injury anxiety. Athl Ther Today 2006;11:57–8.

16. Williams J, Andersen M. Psychosocial antecedents of sport injury: review and critique of the stress and injury model. J Appl Sport Psychol 1998;10(1):5–25.

17. Podlo L, Eklund R. The psychosocial aspects of a return to sport following serious injury: a review of the literature from a self-determination perspective. Psychol Sport Exerc 2007;8:535–66.

18. Gould D, Udry E, Bridges D, et al. Stress sources encountered when rehabilitating from season-ending ski injuries. Sport Psychol 1997;11(4):361–78.

19. Bianco T. Social support and recovery from sport injury: elite skiers share their experiences. Res Q Exerc Sport 2001;72(4):376–88.

20. Podlog L, Eklund R. A longitudinal investigation of competitive athletes' return to sport following serious injury. J Appl Sport Psychol 2006;18(1):44–68.

21. Yang J, Peek-Asa C, Corlette J, et al. Prevalence of and risk factors associated with symptoms of depression in competitive collegiate student athletes. Clin J Sport Med 2007;17(6):481–7.

22. Erlanger D, Kutner K, Barth J, et al. Neuropsychology of sports-related head injury: dementia pugilistica to post concussion syndrome. Clin Neuropsychol 1999;13(2):193–209.

23. Guskiewicz K, Marshall S, Bailes J, et al. Recurrent concussion and risk of depression in retired professional football players. Med Sci Sports Exerc 2007;39:903–9.

24. Hutchison M, Mainwaring L, Comper P, et al. Differential emotional responses of varsity athletes to concussion and musculoskeletal injuries. Clin J Sport Med 2009;19(1):13–9.

25. Mainwaring L, Hutchison M, Bisschop S, et al. Emotional response to sport concussion compared to ACL injury. Brain Inj 2010;24(2):589–97.

26. Granquist M, Hamson-Utley J, Kenow L, et al. Psychosocial strategies for athletic training. Philadelphia, PA: FA Davis; 2014.

27. Chmielewski T, Jones D, Day T, et al. The association of pain and fear of movement/reinjury with function during anterior cruciate ligament reconstruction rehabilitation. J Orthop Sports Phys Ther 2008;38(12):746–53.

28. Kvist J, Sporrstedt K, Good L. Fear of re-injury: a hindrance for returning to sports after anterior cruciate ligament reconstruction. Knee Surg Sports Traumatol Arthrosc 2005;13:393–7.

29. Evans L, Hardy L, Fleming S. Intervention strategies with injured athletes: an action research study. Sport Psychol 2000;14(2):188–206.

30. Walker N, Thatcher J, Lavallee D, et al. The emotional response to athletic injury: re-injury anxiety. In: Lavallee D, Thatcher J, Jones MV, editors. Coping and emotion in sport. Hauppauge (NY): Nova Science Publishers; 2004. p. 91–103.

31. te Wierike S, van der Sluis A, van den Akker-Scheek I, et al. Psychosocial factors influencing the recovery of athletes with anterior cruciate ligament injury: a systematic review. Scand J Med Sci Sports 2013;23(5):527–40.

32. Johnston L, Carroll D. The psychological impact of injury: effects of prior sport and exercise involvement. Br J Sports Med 2000;34:436–9.

33. Arden C, Webster K, Taylor N, et al. Return to sport following anterior cruciate ligament reconstruction surgery: a systematic review and meta-analysis of the state of play. Br J Sports Med 2011;45:596–606.

34. McCullough K, Phelps K, Spindler K, et al. Return to high school- and college-level football after anterior cruciate ligament reconstruction: a Multicenter Orthopaedic Outcomes Network (MOON) cohort study. Am J Sports Med 2012;40(11):2523–9.

35. Flanigan D, Everhart J, Pedroza A, et al. Fear of reinjury (kinesiophobia) and persistent knee symptoms are common factors for lack of return to sport after anterior cruciate ligament reconstruction. Arthroscopy 2013;29(8):1322–9.

36. Kripalani S, LeFevre F, Phillips C, et al. Deficits in communication and information transfer between hospital-based and primary care physicians: implications for patient safety and continuity of care. JAMA 2007;297(8):831–41.
37. Stewart M. Effective physician-patient communication and health outcomes: a review. Can Med Assoc J 1995;152(9):1423.
38. Tongue J, Epps H, Forese L. Communication skills for patient-centered care research-based, easily learned techniques for medical interviews. J Bone Joint Surg 2005;87(3):652–8.
39. Feltz D. The psychology of sports injuries. In: Vinger PE, Hoerner EF, editors. Sports injuries: the unthwarted epidemic. 2nd edition. Boston, MA: John Wright; 1986. p. 336–44.
40. Weiss M, Troxel R. Psychology of the injured athlete. J Athletic Train 1986;21(2): 104–9.
41. Clement D, Granquist M, Arvinen-Barrow M. Psychosocial aspects of athletic injuries as perceived by athletic trainers. J Athletic Train 2013;48(4):512–21.
42. Fisher A, Mullins S, Frye P. Athletic trainers' attitudes and judgments of injured athletes' rehabilitation adherence. J Athletic Train 1993;28(1):43–7.
43. Arvinen-Barrow M. Back to basics: using goal setting to enhance rehabilitation. Sport Exerc Med 2008;37:15–9.
44. Ievleva L, Orlick T. Mental links to enhanced healing: an exploratory study. Sport Psychol 1991;5(1):25–40.
45. Burton D, Naylor S, Holliday B. Goal setting in sport: investigating the goal effectiveness paradox. In: Singer R, Hausenblas H, Janelle C, editors. Handbook of sport psychology. 2nd edition. New York, NY: Wiley; 2001. p. 497–528.
46. Hardy L, Jones J, Gould D. Understanding psychological preparation for sport. Hoboken NJ: John Wiley & Sons Inc; 1996.
47. Hanrahan S, Anderson M. The Routledge handbook of applied sport psychology. Abingdon: Routledge, Taylor & Francis; 2010.
48. Prentice W. Arnheim's principles of athletic training: a competency-based approach. 13th edition. Boston: McGraw Hill; 2013.
49. Ross M, Berger R, Sage G. Effects of stress inoculation training on athletes' post-surgical pain and rehabilitation after orthopedic injury. J Consult Clin Psychol 1996;64:406–10.
50. Potter M, Grove J. Mental skills training ruing rehabilitation: case studies of injured athletes. New Zeal J Physiother 1999;28:24–31.
51. Sordoni C, Hall C, Forwell L. The use of imagery in athletic injury rehabilitation and its relationship to self-efficacy. Physiother Can 2002;54(3):177–85.
52. Vealey R, Greenleaf C. Seeing is believing: understanding and using imagery in sport. 5th edition. New York: McGraw-Hill; 2006.
53. Pavio A. Cognitive and motivational functions of imagery in human performance. Can J Appl Sport Sci 1985;10:22–8.
54. Mortiz S, Hall C, Martin K, et al. What are confident athletes imaging? An examination of image content. Sport Psychol 1996;10:171–9.
55. Rodgrs W, Hall C, Buckholtz E. The effect of an imagery training program on imagery ability, imagery use, and figure skating performance. J Appl Sport Psychol 1991;3:109–25.
56. Pargman D. The use of imagery in the rehabilitation of injured athletes. 3rd edition. Morganton WV: Fitness Information Technology; 2007.
57. Issac A. Mental practice: does it work from the field? Sport Psychol 1992;6:192–8.
58. Hall C, Mack D, Paivio A, et al. Imagery use by athletes: development of the Sport Imagery Questionnaire. Int J Sport Psychol 1998;29(1):73–89.

59. Watt AP, Morris T, Andersen MB. Issues in the development of a measure of imagery ability in sport. J Ment Imagery 2004;28:149–80.

60. Hird J, Landers D, Thomas J, et al. Physical practice is superior to mental practice in enhancing cognitive and motor task performance. J Sport Exerc Psychol 1991;8:281–93.

61. Dawson M, Hamson-Utley J, Hansen R, et al. Examining the effectiveness of psychological strategies on physiologic markers: evidence-based suggestions for holistic care of the athlete. J Athletic Train 2014;49(3):331–7.

62. Williams J, Harris D. Relaxation and energizing techniques for regulation of arousal. In: Williams JM, editor. Applied sport psychology: personal growth to peak performance. 5th edition. Mountain View CA: Mayfield Publishing; 2006. p. 285–305.

63. Jacobson E. Progressive relaxation. Am J Psychol 1987;100(3–4):522–37.

64. Sage G. Introduction to motor behavior: a neuropsychological approach. 2nd edition. London: Addison-Wesley; 1977.

Current and Emerging Rehabilitation for Concussion: A Review of the Evidence

Steven P. Broglio, PhD, ATC[a,b,*], Michael W. Collins, PhD[c],
Richelle M. Williams, MS, ATC[a], Anne Mucha, DPT[c,d],
Anthony P. Kontos, PhD[c]

KEYWORDS

- Concussion - Physical rest - Cognitive rest - Vestibular rehabilitation
- Pharmacologic interventions

KEY POINTS

- Concussion rehabilitation policies are largely consensus based.
- Emerging evidence is suggesting that exercise and cognitive activity in a controlled and prescriptive manner may benefit recovery.
- Additional rehabilitation strategies (eg, vestibular, oculomotor, and pharmacologic) also have mounting evidence and should be incorporated by an appropriately trained professional when appropriate.

INTRODUCTION

The clinical signs and symptoms of sport concussion have long been recognized as[1,2] brought about by an extrinsic force applied directly or indirectly to the head or body.[3] Much of the scientific literature surrounding this injury has focused on injury incidence,[4] assessment tools,[5,6] and recovery patterns among athletes.[7] Absent from the literature are reviews of empirical studies assessing the effectiveness of different rehabilitation approaches for concussed patients. Therefore, this article reviews and evaluates the evidence supporting consensus-based standard of care (eg, physical and cognitive rest) and emerging, targeted (eg, vestibular, oculomotor, exertional, pharmacologic) rehabilitation approaches for concussion based on an evolving model of clinical concussion care.[8]

[a] School of Kinesiology, University of Michigan, Ann Arbor, MI, USA; [b] University of Michigan Injury Center, Ann Arbor, MI, USA; [c] UPMC Sports Medicine Concussion Program, Department of Orthopaedic Surgery, University of Pittsburgh, Pittsburgh, PA, USA; [d] UPMC Centers for Rehab Services, UPMC, Pittsburgh, PA, USA
* Corresponding author. 401 Washtenaw Avenue, Ann Arbor, MI 48109.
E-mail address: broglio@umich.edu

Clin Sports Med 34 (2015) 213–231
http://dx.doi.org/10.1016/j.csm.2014.12.005   **sportsmed.theclinics.com**
0278-5919/15/$ – see front matter © 2015 Elsevier Inc. All rights reserved.

The concept of physical and cognitive rest as the cornerstone of concussion management was developed by the International Concussion in Sport Group and currently states, "The cornerstone of concussion management is physical and cognitive rest until the acute symptoms resolve and then a graded program of exertion prior to medical clearance and return to play."[3] The rationale for rest asserts that during the acute (1–7 days, possibly longer in youth) postinjury period of increased metabolic demand and limited adenosine triphosphate reserves, nonessential activity draws oxygen and glycogen away from injured neurons. The Concussion in Sport Group recommendation has been interpreted by many clinicians to mean that all concussed athletes should be restricted from all physical and cognitive activity until symptoms resolve, at which point, the athlete could be cleared to begin a return to play progression. This "shut-down" or "dark-closet" approach following concussion is wrought with potential pitfalls for patients, including hyperawareness of symptoms, somatization, social isolation, and other potential comorbid concerns. Citing the risk for prolonged and exacerbated symptoms that may not be directly related to the concussive injury, other medical organizations have recommended that athletes be permitted to engage in limited physical and cognitive activity so long as it does not worsen symptoms.[9]

These 2 perspectives regarding strict rest versus physical and cognitive activity as tolerated are seemingly at odds with each other, in part because there is no agreed on definition of what constitutes rest following a concussion in the literature. Such recommendations are also limited because they do not take into account the individualized nature of the injury, potential risk factors that may influence outcomes, and differential responses to recovery. Moreover, and most importantly, there are no known prospective randomized control trials (RCTs) evaluating rest in concussed athletes immediately following a concussion.[10] In fact, the evidence for physical and cognitive rest is limited, relying on observational studies and studies of patients from sports medicine clinics during the subacute stage.[11,12] With a dearth of literature to support clinical guidelines, expert consensus has been used in its place.

The premise that rest is the most effective management strategy for all concussed patients assumes that all concussions are alike, yet concussion recovery is known to be influenced by several modifying factors including sex,[13] concussion history,[14] and age.[15] Even for injuries occurring within these populations, concussions manifest in varied symptoms (eg, headache, dizziness, fogginess), cognitive (eg, memory, reaction time, processing speed),[16] psychological (eg, depression, anxiety),[16] and vestibular (eg, dizziness, imbalance, gait, vestibulo-ocular)[17] impairments. As such, this highly individualized injury results in a varied injury presentation, indicating no single rehabilitation strategy will be effective for all patients following concussion necessitating distinct treatment.[8]

PHYSICAL REST

Declines in neurocognitive function and motor control and increases in self-report symptoms following concussion are well documented.[5,18] Among the most commonly reported symptoms are headache, dizziness, and confusion immediately following a concussion.[19–25] Other research has reported increased rates of depression and fatigue among the same cohort.[26] Between 80% and 90% of concussed individuals will return to preinjury levels of functioning within 2 weeks without intervention, but a small percentage (2.5%) will remain symptomatic 45 days after injury, despite resolution of other objective measures (eg, neurocognitive and balance assessments).[27] Therefore, management of athletes falling within and outside the range of normal recovery may require different approaches.

Evidence for Physical Rest

Consensus supporting physical rest recommendations is partly predicated on risk management and animal studies demonstrating impaired recovery with the early onset of physical activity. Although secondary to restricting activity to facilitate recovery, restricting physical activity to reduce risk for a second injury has broad support as the sole means to eliminate Second Impact Syndrome.[28] Even in the absence of a catastrophic outcome, animal models show metabolic dysfunction in the days immediately following injury[1,29] with an increased energy demand within the cerebral tissue as ion imbalances are returned to preinjury levels. During this time, the risk for second injury seems to be highest[23] and an additional injury sustained shortly after the first increases recovery time and impairs the ability to learn among rodents.[30] Similar metabolic dysfunction findings among concussed athletes were reported by Vagnozzi and colleagues.[31] That is, altered cerebral metabolism lasting up to 30 days was documented using magnetic resonance spectroscopy imaging in concussed athletes and up to 45 days in those sustaining a second injury before resolution of the first.[32]

In addition, subsequent injury risk and prolonged recovery brought about by sport participation, unrestricted physical activity in a controlled and safe environment during the acute recovery stage, may be detrimental. For example, rats exposed to a fluid percussion injury and provided unrestricted running wheel access within the first 6 days of injury showed poorer performance on a cognitive task (ie, Morris water maze) compared with similarly injured rats that were restricted from activity until day 14 after injury.[33] In addition, a review of medical records from 159 concussed patients found that those returning to play before concussion symptom resolution reported worsening concussion-related symptoms.[34] The mechanistic underpinnings explaining these findings are not entirely clear, but it is possible that early exercise may draw energy (ie, glycogen) away from the brain and inhibit the recovery process.

Evidence for Physical Activity

The evidence supporting physical activity following concussion is sparse, but other medical literature suggests that withholding injured, but nonconcussed athletes from exercise increases reports of depression, anxiety, and lower self-esteem when evaluated both at the time of injury and 8 weeks later.[35] Injured (nonconcussed) high school athletes missing a minimum of 3 weeks of athletic participation also showed higher rates of depression than noninjured athletes. The authors indicated that high levels of athletic identity partly explained the finding.[36] Moreover, onset of migraine has been shown to occur in patients with limited or minimal physical activity.[37] Ultimately, removing an athlete from sport may increase the risk for depression and other concussionlike symptoms to develop, yet the point at which an athlete can begin physical activity following concussion is unclear.

In the single human study evaluating exercise shortly after concussion, 95 concussed student-athletes retrospectively self-reported physical and cognitive activity in the 30 days following injury and compared the findings to a neurocognitive assessment. Each athlete was categorized into 1 of 5 groups ranging from "no school or exercise activity" to "school activity and participation in sports games" and completed a computerized neurocognitive assessment for both cognitive functioning and self-report symptoms. The results indicated that athletes engaging in a medium level of physical and cognitive activity (ie, school activity and light activity at home, such as slow jogging or mowing the lawn) performed better on the neurocognitive test than those with no physical and cognitive activity and those reporting the highest levels of physical and cognitive activity.[38] These findings should be cautiously interpreted however, because the physical and cognitive activity was self-report recall by the injured athlete. In addition, it is not known at what point after the injury the athletes elected to begin physical activity. Coupled with the previously discussed animal work, this investigation set the groundwork to suggest that unrestricted exercise in the immediate acute phase of concussion recovery may increase the risk of subsequent injury and/or delay recovery, yet some level of exercise may be beneficial to the recovery process once the athlete has moved beyond the acute injury stage.

When dealing with athletes continuing to experience concussion-like symptoms beyond the acute injury stage, stronger literature is available showing the benefit of physical activity as a means to mitigate symptom reports. Leddy and colleagues[39] implemented a graded return to activity protocol on 6 concussed athletes that had been symptomatic for a minimum of 6 weeks (mean 19 weeks) following a concussive event. Once enrolled, the athletes were monitored for an additional 2 weeks, wherein there was no change in their symptom reports. They then began an exercise protocol 5 to 6 days a week with intensity monitored by heart rate. After 6 weeks of the intervention, the athletes had a significant decrease in their symptom reports and were able to return to sport. Interestingly, a concussed nonathlete group completed an identical protocol, but did not show the same decline in symptom reports as the athlete cohort. A follow-up investigation enrolled 91 participants that had been experiencing symptoms following a concussion for a minimum of 3 weeks. Each participant completed a baseline graded exercise test, whereby 26 were able to reach maximum exertion. These individuals were determined to be experiencing symptoms related to something other than concussion, whereas 35 of the remaining 65 continued with the same heart rate–based exercise protocol described above. A return to full functioning by means of the exercise protocol was achieved in 77% of the subset (n = 27).[40]

Exercise has been proven to be a powerful modality for cognitive health,[41] but the implementation of postconcussion exercise should be carefully considered relative to the time from injury. The limited literature available to date suggests that athletes experiencing symptoms in the acute stage of injury should avoid full sport participation to avoid secondary injury as well as exercise in a controlled environment because it may increase recovery time. Animal and retrospective human studies, however, suggest that athletes continuing to report symptoms beyond the acute stage of injury may benefit from moderate levels of exercise. Last, those athletes that continue to report concussion-related symptoms well beyond the acute stage of injury may benefit from a progressively intensive exercise protocol to return them to their sport.

COGNITIVE REST AND ACADEMIC ACCOMMODATIONS

Cognitive impairment following concussion is common among student-athletes and cognitive rest has been suggested to enhance recovery. The cognitive rest theory is based on the premise that increasing cognitive activities following concussion will increase symptom recovery time and prolong recovery. Cognitive rest includes the reduction of brain stimulating activities (eg, television, video games, school work, reading, and writing) and, despite the limited data to support the use of cognitive rest, it is widely recommended in consensus statements and concussion guidelines.[3,9,42–45]

To date, few studies have evaluated cognitive rest; however, these studies have found that increased cognitive activity does delay symptom recovery. Moser and colleagues[11] studied 49 high school and collegiate athletes prescribed a minimum of a week of cognitive and physical rest. Both before and after rest periods, individuals performed the ImPACT and cognitive testing measures. The study concluded with a period of cognitive and physical rest with individuals showing increased performance on the ImPACT and cognitive testing as well as decreased symptom reporting. Similarly, Brown and colleagues[12] studied 335 patients (mean age, 15 years) on level of cognitive activities between clinical visits, finding that longer concussion recovery time was related to higher cognitive activity levels. Indeed, those participating in the lowest 50% of cognitive activity were completely asymptomatic within 100 to 150 days of injury, whereas those engaging in the third and fourth quartiles of cognitive active took up to 300 and 500 days to recover, respectively.

School is a major component of a student's life, requiring the attainment of new knowledge, development of academic skills, and diligent work to complete assignments and prepare for examinations. To be successful in academic endeavors, students must engage in classroom learning requiring attention, material memory recall, critical thinking, and problem-solving. Students who sustain a sports-related concussion (SRC) may also experience physical, mental, behavioral, and social changes that impact their daily life and threaten their ability to learn and succeed academically.[46] Limiting school activity is one mechanism that affords the injured athlete time to mitigate concussion-related symptoms.

Despite limited research on cognitive load following concussion, it has been suggested that some concussed students may benefit from excused or reduced academics (eg, classroom attendance, homework, examinations) immediately following injury.[47–49] Returning to academic work while symptomatic may cause symptoms to worsen, resulting in a decline in academic performance.[48,50] Although there are more formal accommodations available for long-term or prolonged cases, temporary and targeted accommodations during the acute recovery time is an easy tool to assist a student's return to the classroom.[47] Temporary accommodations may include, but are not limited to, excused absences, lighter homework, breaks during the day, starting later or ending the school day earlier, and extended examination or homework dates.[49] Once the athlete no longer reports concussion-related symptoms, a transition period to partial and then full days is recommended.[51]

Requiring a student-athlete to attend school immediately following a concussion may place him or her in a compromised academic position. Concussed student-athletes engaging in moderate to intense cognitive activity may exacerbate symptoms,[12] resulting in incomplete school work, making excused absences important to the recovery process. During this period, a time extension to complete academic assignments including homework and examinations allows the student-athlete to make up missed schoolwork and take their time with completion of assignments. Implementing delayed testing or project due dates can help the student maintain good academic standing without the penalty of decreased scores. Temporary accommodations such as these are commonly implemented quickly and without burdensome paperwork. To ensure these tools are available, the concussion management team should prearrange their use with school personnel as part of the concussion management plan before the athletic season.

Those individuals experiencing a prolonged concussion recovery or those with recurrent injuries may need additional testing to better accommodate or intervene with school as needed.[51] In some cases, implementing an individualized academic plan can help with the management of accommodations. If a student-athlete is having symptoms or displays challenges greater than 3 weeks, a 504 Plan may be implemented.[47] A 504 Plan refers to the proper section of the Rehabilitation Act that provides medical need accommodations. In order for formal accommodations to be implemented, the student would have to display mental impairments that limit greater than one major life activity.[52] Clinicians may also consider an Individualized Education

Plan (IEP) for those with prolonged concussion recovery. An IEP allows for the school personnel to collaborate with the physician, student-athlete, and parents to create a plan that will best help that student receive special education.[53] Both IEPs and 504 Plans require extensive medical documentation and are a more permanent measure that are embedded into the school system documents, but allow for changes to the student-athlete's academic plan for classroom success.

Despite consensus for cognitive rest, it is important to note that prolonged cognitive rest and reduction of school events have the potential to exacerbate symptoms or cause negative mental health issues. Depression, behavioral issues, and social issues have been shown to increase following a concussion as well as many other injuries when the student-athlete is eliminated from team activities, school events, and social outings.[54] Decreasing school attendance and other social activities can negatively impact some student-athletes and prevent them from going through proper injury-coping mechanisms. Decreased school attendance can also add an increased burden and sense of anxiety to the student-athlete because they are not attending school nor completing school assignments. The mental image of being behind in academics can create a highly anxious environment for student-athletes, especially those who already place high priority on increased academic achievement. Ultimately, the medical team, in conjunction with a trained professional, should balance the neurocognitive and behavioral accommodations of the concussed student-athlete in a way that restricts cognitive activities that trigger or introduce symptom exacerbation, but allow for him or her to become involved in school activities again.

VESTIBULAR AND OCULOMOTOR REHABILITATION

In a new clinical model of SRC care, researchers have suggested that oculomotor and vestibular symptoms and impairment may constitute unique clinical subtypes of SRC—along with cognitive fatigue, anxiety-mood, cervical, and posttraumatic migraine (PTM).[8] These clinical subtypes of concussion, which can occur concurrently or independently, require targeted therapies and treatments to be managed most effectively.[8] For example, an athlete with an oculomotor concussion subtype will benefit most from vision and oculomotor-specific therapies. Without such targeted intervention strategies, an athlete may experience an unnecessarily prolonged recovery from SRC. In a prospective study of recovery times following SRC, researchers reported that 17% of athletes experience prolonged recovery lasting greater than 3 weeks.[55] The identification of specific clinical subtypes of concussion together with the application of targeted treatments and rehabilitation strategies will yield the best clinical outcomes for athletes with SRC. Two clinical subtypes that have been associated with poor clinical outcomes, but that may be amenable to rehabilitation and treatment interventions, are vestibular and oculomotor.

Vestibular and Oculomotor Impairment and Symptoms

Vestibular and oculomotor impairment and symptoms occur in approximately 60% of athletes following SRC.[17] The vestibular system plays an integral role in balance function and in maintaining visual and spatial orientation. Sensory information from each inner ear is used to inform the adjustment of eye movements for clear, stable vision and to adjust muscle reactions of the head and body for balance and gait. Vestibular impairment and dysfunction may involve either the peripheral or the central structures of the vestibulospinal system and may result in disequilibrium and impaired balance.[56] In contrast, dizziness, vertigo, blurred/unstable vision, discomfort in busy environments, and nausea often occur with disruption to the vestibulo-ocular system.[56]

Vestibular symptoms at the time of injury may predict prolonged recovery following SRC. In fact, Lau and colleagues[25] reported that on-field dizziness was the only significant predictor of a prolonged recovery (>21 days) following SRC. This expression of post-SRC dizziness acutely may be the result of disruption to the vestibulo-ocular and gaze stability systems at the time of the injury.

Similar to vestibular dysfunction, impairment in oculomotor control and visual dysfunction are observed frequently following SRC.[57–61] Ciuffreda and colleagues[62] indicated that visual dysfunction involving accommodation, version and vergence, strabismus, and cranial nerve palsy occurred following mild traumatic brain injury (mTBI). Symptoms attributed to poor oculomotor function may include blurred vision, diplopia, difficulty reading, eyestrain, headache, reading difficulties, and problems with visual scanning. Vestibular and oculomotor impairment and symptoms are prevalent following SRC and may play a role in prolonged recovery and related clinical outcomes. Therefore, vestibular rehabilitation and vision therapy interventions are presented and discussed that can be used with athletes experiencing vestibular and oculomotor impairment and symptoms following SRC.

Vestibular Rehabilitation Interventions

There are many different types of vestibular rehabilitation interventions that may be implemented to mitigate vestibular symptoms and dysfunction following SRC. Among the most common vestibular issues following SRC are benign paroxysmal positional vertigo (BPPV), vestibulo-ocular reflex (VOR) impairment, visual motion sensitivity, balance dysfunction, cervicogenic dizziness, and exercise-induced dizziness. **Table 1** summarizes these and other vestibular problems along with targeted therapeutic interventions. It is important to note that these interventions should be performed by licensed physical therapists specializing in vestibular rehabilitation.

Benign paroxysmal positional vertigo is the most common disorder of the vestibular system and can occur posttraumatically after SRC. In BPPV, small calcium carbonate crystals (otoconia), which are normally housed in the otolith organs of the inner ear, become dislodged and relocate to one or more of the adjacent semicircular canals. With head movement in the plane of the affected semicircular canal, the otoconia shift position and create a false excitatory stimulus and resultant vertigo. Reproduction of vertigo and a characteristic nystagmus pattern during positional testing (Dix-Hallpike and Roll Test) are necessary to diagnose BPPV. Canalith repositioning maneuvers, designed to shift the displaced otoconia out of the affected semicircular canal, is the treatment of choice for BPPV.[63]

Gaze stability refers to the ability to maintain visual focus while the head is moving. Although gaze stability is mediated by different vestibular and ocular motor systems depending on the velocity and context of the task, the VOR is the primary mechanism for maintaining eye position during head movement. The VOR is a fast-acting reflex that keeps the eyes stable by generating ocular movements precisely in proportion, but opposite in direction, from the head motion. In sport, where rapid acceleration and high-velocity movement necessitate quick visual responses, intact VOR functioning is particularly important. When the VOR is impaired, visual blurring, dizziness, poor visual focus, and oscillopsia may occur with head motion. The responses of the VOR can be adapted through exercise designed to induce movement of a visual image on the retina. This motion, inducing retinal slip, is the primary error signal that drives adaptation of the VOR. Thus, vestibular physical therapy exercises for VOR adaptation require patients to maintain visual focus on a target while moving their head. VOR adaptation exercises are manipulated in multiple ways to gain maximal benefit,

Table 1
Common interventions for vestibular impairment following sport-related concussion

Impairment	Cause	Symptoms	Associated Problems/Risk Factors	Physical Therapy Treatment
Benign paroxysmal positional vertigo[63]	Mechanical disruption in the vestibular labyrinth (end organ). Otoconia from otoliths become dislodged and displace in semicircular canal	Vertigo with changes in head position	Older age High impact forces	Canalith repositioning maneuvers
VOR impairment[80]	Disrupted function in the VOR pathways, peripherally or centrally	Dizziness	Labyrinthine concussion	Gaze stability training
Visual motion sensitivity[90]	Impaired central processing/ integration of vestibular information with visual and other sensory information	Dizziness	Posttraumatic migraine Anxiety	Graded exposure to visually stimulating environments Virtual reality Optokinetic stimulation
Impaired postural control[91]	Disruption/damage to vestibular-spinal reflex pathways, peripherally or centrally	Impaired balance, particularly with: • Vision and/or somatosensation reduced • Cognitive dual/task demand	Common early finding after concussion; typically resolves before other vestibular deficits	Balance rehabilitation strategies Sensory organization training Divided attention training Dynamic balance training
Cervicogenic dizziness[92,93]	Cervical injury results in abnormal afferent input to CNS; mismatch with other sensory information	Dizziness, related to cervical movement/posture Imbalance Impaired oculomotor control	Cervical pathologic abnormality Cervicogenic headaches	Manual therapy for cervical spine Balance training Oculomotor training
Exercise-induced dizziness[94]	Inadequate central response to cardiovascular and vestibular/ocular demands of exercise	Dizziness with movement-related cardiovascular exercise	• VOR/gaze stability impairment • Visual motion sensitivity • Autonomic dysregulation	Progressive dynamic exertion exercise program

including varying target size and complexity, postures, duration, direction, amplitude, and velocity.

Visual motion sensitivity refers to an increased sense of disorientation, dizziness, or postural instability in situations with visual and vestibular conflict. It is thought to arise from inability of the central nervous system (CNS) to effectively integrate sensory information, particularly vestibular information, creating overreliance on vision. Patients with visual motion sensitivity become particularly symptomatic when exposed to visually disorienting stimuli or environments, such as malls, grocery stores, or even busy patterns. Visual motion sensitivity has also been described as "visual vertigo," "space and motion discomfort," and "visual vestibular mismatch" in the literature. Visual motion sensitivity has been reported in patients following peripheral vestibular disorders[64] and in those with migraine[65] and anxiety.[66] It has also recently been recognized in patients following SRC.[17] Treatment of visual motion sensitivity involves gradual and systematic exposure to provocative stimuli to habituate the abnormal responses. Because treatment of visual motion sensitivity has the potential to exacerbate symptoms from concussion, intervention should be introduced in a step-by-step progression that is carefully monitored by a trained vestibular therapist.

Restoring postural control, or balance, is an area of focus for vestibular rehabilitation following SRC.[67–69] Because sensory organization is often impaired[70,71] early after concussion, training the ability to effectively alternate between using visual, somatosensory, and vestibular information for postural control is a key component of balance retraining. Graded exercises for sensory organization deficits involve manipulation of these 3 sensory systems. Examples of sensory organization training activities include performing tasks with eyes closed, while turning the head, with narrowed base of support, on an uneven or soft surface. In addition to sensory organization issues, several studies have shown patients following mTBI have greater difficulty maintaining balance under conditions of divided attention.[72–74] Therefore, dual task condition practice and dynamic balance activities may also be incorporated into vestibular rehabilitation.

Although dizziness is most often attributed to vestibular system dysfunction, it may also arise from other impairment following SRC, which may be responsive to intervention. In cervicogenic dizziness, pathologic abnormality in the cervical spine creates abnormal muscle activity in the deep layers of the upper cervical spine responsible for providing proprioceptive input to the CNS. Dizziness is thought to occur because of the mismatch between aberrant cervical proprioceptive information in relation to vestibular and visual inputs. Because this cervical afferent information also participates in reflex activity for postural control and eye movements, imbalance and impaired eye movements may occur in addition to dizziness. Management of cervicogenic dizziness is directed toward therapies that treat the underlying cervical spine injury to normalize proprioceptive input with visual and vestibular information, along with treatment of any additional balance or oculomotor impairment through targeted exercises (Treleaven 2011).

Last, following concussion, dizziness may arise with exertional activity.[75] In a study of soldiers following blast-related concussion, exercise-induced dizziness was categorized as one type of dizziness typically seen by physical therapists in vestibular rehabilitation. Although there are no studies that confirm the cause of exercise-induced dizziness, the authors postulate that inadequate response of the CNS to combined cardiovascular and vestibular/visual demand may be responsible. Anecdotally, it was found in the authors' clinic that stationary cardiovascular activities at high levels of exertion (eg, stationary cycling) rarely cause dizziness, whereas cardiovascular activity maintaining similar levels of exertion, when combined with motion (eg, forward/backward line drills), often produces significant levels of dizziness. Clearly, more research is needed to validate this hypothesis. Treatment of individuals with exercise-induced symptoms is controversial; however, preliminary evidence suggests that graded exercise may be useful in modifying these postconcussive symptoms when chronic.[39,76]

The value of vestibular rehabilitation in managing individual vestibular conditions is well documented. A *Cochrane Review*[77] concluded that there is moderate to strong evidence for efficacy of vestibular rehabilitation in improving VOR impairment and balance deficits due to peripheral vestibular dysfunction, and for the use of canalith repositioning maneuvers performed by vestibular therapists in the management of BPPV. Dizziness due to migraine as well as patients with central vestibular dysfunction has been shown in studies to improve with vestibular physical therapy intervention (Whitney and colleagues, 2000; Brown and colleagues, 2006). Therapies for visual motion sensitivity, such as optokinetic stimulus exposure, have been shown to be effective with peripheral vestibular disorders (Pavlou 2013). Several studies have investigated the efficacy of physical therapy treatment of the cervical spine for cervicogenic dizziness (Malmstrom 2007, Heidenreich 2008, Reid 2008), including a recent RCT (Reid 2014) demonstrating significant reduction in intensity and frequency of cervicogenic dizziness with 2 different manual therapy techniques over placebo. Although vestibular therapies have been shown to be beneficial in the treatment of various vestibular-related impairments, the evidence for using vestibular physical therapy for impairment attributed to SRC is limited and consists primarily of retrospective, cross-sectional, and small cohort studies.

A recent study by Schneider and colleagues[78] conducted an RCT with a sample of 12- to 30-year-olds with dizziness, neck pain, and/or headache following SRC. After 8 weekly physical therapy sessions consisting of vestibular and cervical spine rehabilitation, subjects in the treatment group were nearly 4 times more likely to be medically cleared when compared with a control group. In a retrospective chart review, Alsalaheen and colleagues[79] examined the response of a population of concussed patients to vestibular physical therapy. Data from 114 patients referred for vestibular rehabilitation following concussion demonstrated a significant treatment effect for 15 different measures of dizziness severity, balance confidence, gait, and static/dynamic balance. Gottshall and Hoffer[75] assessed computerized VOR and gaze stability measures in 82 military individuals who experienced blast-related mTBI. Impairment was significant at the time of initial evaluation, but returned to normative levels after 4 to 12 weeks of vestibular physical therapy. Hoffer and colleagues[80] examined the effect of vestibular rehabilitation in a population of 58 active duty military individuals with postconcussive dizziness. They found that after a 6- to 8-week vestibular rehabilitation program, patients had improved with respect to symptoms of dizziness, perception of balance function, and measures of VOR function. However, the effectiveness of vestibular rehabilitation differed based on type of posttraumatic dizziness. Specifically, patients with PTM-associated dizziness were most responsive to treatment (84%) in contrast with the spatial disorientation group (27%).

Vision Therapy

Most oculomotor problems following SRC, such as convergence insufficiency, accommodative insufficiency, impaired version movements, and minor ocular misalignments, may be managed conservatively with vision therapy.[57] However, in rare instances, surgical/medical intervention by an ophthalmologist or neuro-ophthalmologist may be warranted for complex diplopia, strabismus that is due to muscle paralysis or nerve palsy, or other concurrent ocular-health issues. Typically, vision therapy involves vision exercises using eye patches, penlights, mirrors, lenses, prisms, and other nonsurgical interventions to improve the function of the ocular muscles.

Despite anecdotal evidence for the effectiveness of vision therapy following SRC, there is limited empirical support for vision therapy in the literature. However, a 2011 *Cochrane Review* of RCTs for nonsurgical intervention for convergence insufficiency, and another RCT by Scheiman and colleagues for treatment of accommodative insufficiency, pointed to the effectiveness of vision therapy in children in managing these 2 conditions.[81,82] Although empirical support for oculomotor and vision-related therapies following SRC is limited and does not include any RCTs, emerging evidence supports the effectiveness of visual exercises for specific oculomotor problems. A retrospective study by Ciuffreda and colleagues[62] examined patients with mTBI who were enrolled in a vision therapy program consisting of combined vergence, version, and accommodative exercises. They reported that 90% of patients improved markedly or completely in symptoms and subjective reports of enhanced reading at a 2 – to –3-month follow-up. In a recent study involving 12 subjects following mTBI, Thiagarajan and Ciuffreda[83] demonstrated that an oculomotor training program targeting the version, vergence, and accommodation components of the ocular motor system significantly improved the amplitudes of vergence and accommodation, accuracy of saccadic eye movements, and overall reading.

PHARMACOLOGIC INTERVENTIONS

It has been reported that as much as 89% of clinicians manage symptoms of athletes with SRC using over-the-counter (OTC) or prescription medications.[84] The most common interventions involve OTC medications such as nonsteroidal anti-inflammatory drugs and acetaminophen. However, many other prescription pharmacologic interventions are used with athletes who are not following a normal recovery trajectory (ie, recovered within 10–14 days) following SRC. Research indicates that pharmacologic treatments usually begin at approximately 10 days after injury.[42] As with vestibular and oculomotor therapies, pharmacologic interventions are most effective when they target specific clinical subtypes of SRC. For example, an athlete with a primary cognitive-fatigue subtype following SRC may be prescribed a neurostimulant such as amantadine. In addition to cognitive fatigue, other clinical subtypes that are amenable to pharmacologic treatment include PTM and anxiety/mood.[3,8] In addition, sleep-related issues are often treated using pharmacologic interventions. It is important to acknowledge that there is still no US Food and Drug Administration–approved pharmacologic treatment for SRC. As such, all pharmacologic interventions discussed later involve off-label use of medications that were approved for other primary purposes. Moreover, each medication discussed may involve side effects that warrant close monitoring from prescribing clinicians. In addition, the use of certain medications, such as neurostimulants, may be in violation of the medication and performance enhancement policies of specific sport governing bodies; thus, proper documentation is very important.

Targeted Pharmacologic Interventions: Matching Treatments to Clinical Subtypes

Cognitive fatigue is a commonly targeted clinical subtype for pharmacologic intervention. Athletes with this subtype experience difficulty concentrating, memory problems, attentional issues, decreased vigor, and headaches that worsen throughout the day. These symptoms are often treated effectively with the use of a neurostimulant. The most commonly used neurostimulant is amantadine, with 10% of clinicians reporting that they prescribe amantadine to athletes following SRC.[84] There is some empirical evidence that amantadine, a dopaminergic neurostimulant primarily purposed as a antiviral medication, can improve cognitive-fatigue symptoms and memory in athletes experiencing prolonged recovery following SRC.[85] Other neurostimulants that can be used to treat athletes with cognitive fatigue include methylphenidate, Adderall, and atomoxetine. There is some evidence of the effectiveness of methylphenidate on improving processing speed in moderate TBI (eg, [86]), but not in athletes with SRC. Of note, some athletes may already be taking these medications for attention deficit hyperactivity disorder and related conditions, thereby necessitating close monitoring from clinicians; medications may need to be adjusted during their recovery period.

Some athletes may develop anxiety or mood issues as a direct result of an SRC or secondary to the injury recovery process with its concomitant frustrations and feelings of isolation and loss of control.[16] Other athletes may have pre-existing anxiety/mood issues before injury that may be exacerbated following an SRC. Regardless of its underlying cause, anxiety and mood issues following SRC can be treated with tricyclic antidepressants (eg, amitriptyline). In fact, tricyclic antidepressants are used by up to 23% of clinicians in treating young athletes with SRC.[84] It is likely that this relatively high percentage of clinicians prescribing tricyclic antidepressants is due in part to its use across multiple clinical subtypes, including anxiety and mood, sleep, and PTM. Other common medications used for athletes in the anxiety and mood clinical subtype include selective serotonin reuptake inhibitors (SSRI) and selective norepinephrine reuptake inhibitors. There is some anecdotal evidence that short-term, low-dosage use of certain benzodiazepines such as Klonopin may be effective in athletes with vestibular-related anxiety. Klonopin and other benzodiapenes are also thought to act on neurons in the vestibular nuclei of the brain to decrease vestibular-related symptoms and in turn decrease anxiety. Klonopin can be effective for vestibular-related migraines. However, Klonopin can result in elevated anxiety and sleep disruption in some athletes and its use should be monitored closely.

The symptoms of PTM include headache, nausea, photo-sensitivity or phono-sensitivity, and dizziness. These symptoms have been associated with prolonged recovery and impairment following SRC.[87] Clinicians may use a variety of pharmacologic interventions to treat the symptoms of PTM, including tricyclic and SSRI antidepressants, anticonvulsants (eg, topiramate, gabapentin, valproic acid), or β-blockers. In addition, triptans (eg, Imitrex, Maxalt) are often prescribed as abortive medications for PTM. Despite anecdotal evidence regarding the effectiveness of these treatments, there are no empirical studies of the effectiveness of these medications in athletes with SRC.

There is often a sleep overlay that permeates across each clinical subtype of SRC. Consequently, clinicians often prescribe OTC and prescription sleep medications for athletes with persistent sleep disruptions following SRC. After all, if an athlete is not sleeping well following an SRC, it will be difficult for that athlete to recover. The most commonly used sleep medication is melatonin with one-fifth of clinicians reporting that they prescribe melatonin to athletes with sleep disruptions following SRC.[84] Melatonin together with basic sleep hygiene can help regulate circadian rhythms and promote better sleep-wake cycling.[88,89] Other medications used to improve sleep disruption in athletes following SRC include antidepressants (eg, amitriptyline, trazodone) and nonbenzodiazepine hypnotics (eg, Ambien, Lunesta).[89]

SUMMARY AND RECOMMENDATIONS

Despite limited empirical support, physical and cognitive rest have been deemed essential components of initial concussion management and treatment. Such recommendations have been developed by consensus and introduced by the International Concussion in Sport Group in 2008. Since that time, there has been limited empirical work evaluating the efficacy of physical and cognitive rest protocols. Some research suggests that prescribed physical and cognitive rest in the acute stage of concussion may be of benefit to some athletes. However, other studies have indicated that an early return to light to moderate physical activity may be effective for other athletes following concussion. The heterogeneous nature of concussion renders a universal prescription of strict rest for all concussed athletes an ineffective strategy. As such, strict rest extending beyond the acute injury stage may result in the athlete developing concussionlike symptoms that are unrelated to the injury (eg, anxiety, migraine, sleep disorders) and may complicate injury management, which may in turn lead to psychological and other concurrent problems. Student-athletes who are unable to attend or participate in academics to the fullest may benefit from a reduced cognitive load following injury, with a graduated return to academics that does not exacerbate symptoms. Reduction of cognitive load requires a coordinated effort between the medical and school academic support staff with short-term or long-term academic accommodations. Any accommodations may be lifted once a complete academic schedule can be completed without symptom exacerbation, at which time a return to play protocol be undertaken.

Sport-related concussions can involve several different clinical subtypes that warrant a comprehensive clinical assessment and subsequent targeted treatment and rehabilitation strategies. Recent advances in screening for vestibular and oculomotor impairment and symptoms (eg, Mucha and colleagues[17]) have revealed that many athletes experience these issues following SRC. Research also suggests that athletes with these issues often have longer recovery times and more pronounced impairment and symptoms following SRC.[25] In response to these findings, vestibular and vision therapists have begun to apply specific rehabilitation interventions to enhance the recovery process for those athletes with vestibular or oculomotor impairment and symptoms following SRC. Initial empirical evidence indicates that these vestibular and oculomotor interventions may be useful in mitigating these issues and enhancing the recovery of athletes with SRC. However, additional research regarding which interventions are most effective for each type of impairment and symptoms as well as the optimal number and length of therapeutic sessions needed to obtain the desired effect is warranted.

Most clinicians use some sort of OTC or prescription pharmacologic intervention to help manage lingering symptoms and impairment following SRC.[84] It is clear from clinical experience that when pharmacologic treatments are matched appropriately with patients' clinical subtypes and symptoms, they can be an effective intervention. However, there is some overlap for the effectiveness of certain pharmacologic interventions across more than one clinical subtype. Most pharmacologic treatments are implemented in patients with lingering (10–14 + days) or chronic (3 + months) symptoms and impairments. It is atypical for a patient to be prescribed a medication in the acute and subacute phases following a concussion. This "wait-and-see" approach may result in missed opportunities for effective early pharmacologic intervention following SRC. However, researchers have yet to determine how soon after injury the preceding pharmacologic treatments should be implemented to have the greatest therapeutic effect. In fact, it has been suggested that clinicians could accelerate recovery for some patients if pharmacologic treatments were implemented earlier in the injury process. In addition, researchers need to explore the effectiveness of various dosage levels, treatment regimens, and administration methods in patients following concussion.

This review was conceived to evaluate the evidence supporting current and emerging rehabilitation approaches for sport concussion. Consensus opinion for prescribed physical and cognitive rest is the most common rehabilitation approach for patients with concussion. However, more active and targeted rehabilitation strategies including vestibular and oculomotor rehabilitation and pharmacologic interventions have emerging evidence supporting their use. Ultimately, there is limited empirical support for the rehabilitation strategies discussed in this article, necessitating additional research on their effectiveness following concussion. This research should use multisite, RCT research designs to better elucidate the specific effects of individual interventions. In addition, future research should use comprehensive outcome assessments and targeted rehabilitation strategies that account for the heterogeneous nature of this injury.

REFERENCES

1. Giza CC, Hovda DA. The neurometabolic cascade of concussion. J Athl Train 2001;36(3):228–35.
2. Giza CC, Hovda DA. The new neurometabolic cascade of concussion. Neurosurgery 2014;75(Suppl 4):S24–33.
3. McCrory P, Meeuwisse WH, Aubry M, et al. Consensus statement on concussion in sport: the 4th International Conference on Concussion in Sport held in Zurich, November 2012. Br J Sports Med 2013;47(5):250–8.
4. National Collegiate Athletic Association. NCAA injury surveillance summary for 15 sports: 1988–1999 through 2003–2004. J Athl Train 2007;42(2):165–320.
5. Broglio SP, Puetz TW. The effect of sport concussion on neurocognitive function, self-report symptoms, and postural control: a meta-analysis. Sports Med 2008; 38(1):53–67.
6. McCrea M, Barr WB, Guskiewicz KM, et al. Standard regression-based methods for measuring recovery after sport-related concussion. J Int Neuropsychol Soc 2005;11:58–69.
7. McCrea M, Guskiewicz KM, Marshall SW, et al. Acute effects and recovery time following concussion in collegiate football players: the NCAA concussion study. JAMA 2003;290(19):2556–63.
8. Collins MW, Kontos AP, Reynolds E, et al. A comprehensive, targeted approach to the clinical care of athletes following sport-related concussion. Knee Surg Sports Traumatol Arthrosc 2014;22(2):235–46.
9. Broglio SP, Cantu RC, Gioia GA, et al. National athletic trainers' association position statement: management of sport concussion. J Athl Train 2014;49(2):245–65.
10. Committee on Sports-Related Concussions in Youth, Board on Children, Youth, and Families, Institute of Medicine, National Research Council. The National Academies Collection: reports funded by National Institutes of Health. In: Graham R, Rivara FP, Ford MA, et al, editors. Sports-related concussions in youth: improving the science, changing the culture. Washington, DC: National Academies Press (US); 2014. Copyright 2014 by the National Academy of Sciences. All rights reserved.
11. Moser RS, Glatts C, Schatz P. Efficacy of immediate and delayed cognitive and physical rest for treatment of sports-related concussion. J Pediatr 2012;161(5): 922–6.

12. Brown NJ, Mannix RC, O'Brien MJ, et al. Effect of cognitive activity level on duration of post-concussion symptoms. Pediatrics 2014;133(2):e299–304.
13. Covassin T, Swanik CB, Sachs M, et al. Sex differences in baseline neuropsychological function and concussion symptoms of collegiate athletes. Br J Sports Med 2006;40(11):923–7 [discussion: 927].
14. Iverson GL, Gaetz M, Lovell MR, et al. Cumulative effects of concussion in amateur athletes. Brain Inj 2004;18(5):433–43.
15. Field M, Collins MW, Lovell MR, et al. Does age play a role in recovery from sports-related concussion? A comparison of high school and collegiate athletes. J Pediatr 2003;142(5):546–53.
16. Kontos AP, Collins M, Russo S. An introduction to sport concussion for the sport psychology consultant. Appl Sport Psyc 2004;16(3):220–35.
17. Mucha A, Collins MW, Elbin RJ, et al. A brief vestibular/ocular motor screening (VOMS) assessment to evaluate concussions: preliminary findings. Am J Sports Med 2014;42(10):2479–86.
18. Belanger HG, Vanderploeg RD. The neuropsychological impact of sports-related concussion: a meta-analysis. J Int Neuropsychol Soc 2005;11:345–57.
19. Collins MW, Field M, Lovell MR, et al. Relationship between postconcussion headache and neuropsychological test performance in high school athletes. Am J Sports Med 2003;31(2):168–73.
20. Collins MW, Iverson GL, Lovell MR, et al. On-field predictors of neuropsychological and symptom deficit following sports-related concussion. Clin J Sport Med 2003;13(4):222–9.
21. Delaney JS, Lacroix VJ, Leclerc S, et al. Concussions among university football and soccer players. Clin J Sport Med 2002;12(6):331–8.
22. Guskiewicz KM, Weaver NL, Padua DA, et al. Epidemiology of concussion in collegiate and high school football players. Am J Sports Med 2000;28(5):643–50.
23. Guskiewicz KM, McCrea M, Marshall SW, et al. Cumulative effects associated with recurrent concussion in collegiate football players: the NCAA concussion study. JAMA 2003;290(19):2549–55.
24. McCrory PR, Ariens M, Berkovic SF. The nature and duration of acute concussive symptoms in Australian football. Clin J Sport Med 2000;10:235–8.
25. Lau BC, Kontos AP, Collins MW, et al. Which on-field signs/symptoms predict protracted recovery from sport-related concussion among high school football players? Am J Sports Med 2011;39(11):2311–8.
26. Eisenberg MA, Meehan WP 3rd, Mannix R. Duration and course of post-concussive symptoms. Pediatrics 2014;133(6):999–1006.
27. McCrea M, Guskiewicz KM, Randolph C, et al. Incidence, clinical course, and predictors of prolonged recovery time following sport-related concussion in high school and college athletes. J Int Neuropsychol Soc 2013;19(1):22–33.
28. Bruce DA, Alavi A, Bilaniuk L, et al. Diffuse cerebral swelling following head injuries in children: the syndrome of "malignant brain edema". J Neurosurg 1981;54(2):170–8.
29. Giza CC, Difiori JP. Pathophysiology of sports-related concussion: an update on basic science and translational research. Sports Health 2011;3(1):46–51.
30. Prins ML, Hales A, Reger M, et al. Repeat traumatic brain injury in the juvenile rat is associated with increased axonal injury and cognitive impairments. Dev Neurosci 2010;32(5–6):510–8.
31. Vagnozzi R, Signoretti S, Cristofori L, et al. Assessment of metabolic brain damage and recovery following mild traumatic brain injury: a multicentre, proton

magnetic resonance spectroscopic study in concussed patients. Brain 2010; 133(11):3232–42.

32. Vagnozzi R, Signoretti S, Tavazzi B, et al. Temporal window of metabolic brain vulnerability to concussion: a pilot H-magnetic resonance spectroscopy study in concussed athletes - part III. Neurosurgery 2008;62(6):1286–95.

33. Griesbach GS, Hovda DA, Molteni R, et al. Voluntary exercise following traumatic brain injury: brain-derived neurotrophic factor upregulation and recovery of function. Neuroscience 2004;125(1):129–39.

34. Carson JD, Lawrence DW, Kraft SA, et al. Premature return to play and return to learn after a sport-related concussion: physician's chart review. Can Fam Physician 2014;60(6):e310, e312–5.

35. Leddy MH, Lambert MJ, Ogles BM. Psychological consequences of athletic injury among high-level competitors. Res Q Exerc Sport 1994;65(4):347–54.

36. Manuel JC, Shilt JS, Curl WW, et al. Coping with sports injuries: an examination of the adolescent athlete. J Adolesc Health 2002;31(5):391–3.

37. Milde-Busch A, Blaschek A, Borggrafe I, et al. Associations of diet and lifestyle with headache in high-school students: results from a cross-sectional study. Headache 2010;50(7):1104–14.

38. Majerske CW, Mihalik JP, Ren D, et al. Concussion in sports: postconcussive activity levels, symptoms, and neurocognitive performance. J Athl Train 2008;43(3): 265–74.

39. Leddy JJ, Kozlowski K, Donnelly JP, et al. A preliminary study of subsymptom threshold exercise training for refractory post-concussion syndrome. Clin J Sport Med 2010;20(1):21–7.

40. Baker JG, Freitas MS, Leddy JJ, et al. Return to full functioning after graded exercise assessment and progressive exercise treatment of postconcussion syndrome. Rehabil Res Pract 2012;2012:705309.

41. Vancampfort D, Probst M, Adriaens A, et al. Changes in physical activity, physical fitness, self-perception and quality of life following a 6-month physical activity counseling and cognitive behavioral therapy program in outpatients with binge eating disorder. Psychiatry Res 2014;219(2):361–6.

42. Giza CC, Kutcher JS, Ashwal S, et al. Summary of evidence-based guideline update: evaluation and management of concussion in sports: report of the guideline development subcommittee of the American Academy of Neurology. Neurology 2013;80(24):2250–7.

43. Halstead ME, Walter KD, Council on Sports Medicine and Fitness. American Academy of Pediatrics. Clinical report–sport-related concussion in children and adolescents. Pediatrics 2010;126(3):597–615.

44. Herring SA, Cantu RC, Guskiewicz KM, et al. Concussion (mild traumatic brain injury) and the team physician: a consensus statement–2011 update. Med Sci Sports Exerc 2011;43(12):2412–22.

45. Harmon KG, Drezner J, Gammons M, et al. American Medical Society for Sports Medicine position statement: concussion in sport. Clin J Sport Med 2013;23(1): 1–18.

46. Mealings M, Douglas J, Olver J. Considering the student perspective in returning to school after TBI: a literature review. Brain Inj 2012;26(10):1165–76.

47. Halstead ME, McAvoy K, Devore CD, et al. Returning to learning following a concussion. Pediatrics 2013;132(5):948–57.

48. Sady MD, Vaughan CG, Gioia GA. School and the concussed youth: recommendations for concussion education and management. Phys Med Rehabil Clin N Am 2011;22(4):701–19.

49. McGrath N. Supporting the student-athlete's return to the classroom after a sport-related concussion. J Athl Train 2010;45(5):492–8.
50. Howell D, Osternig L, Van Donkelaar P, et al. Effects of concussion on attention and executive function in adolescents. Med Sci Sports Exerc 2013;45(6):1030–7.
51. McGrath N, Dinn WM, Collins MW, et al. Post-exertion neurocognitive test failure among student-athletes following concussion. Brain Inj 2013;27(1):103–13.
52. Rehabilitation Act of 1973 amendment 29 U.S.C. § 794 (Section 504). U.S Department of Education; 2012.
53. Piebes SK, Gourley M, Valovich McLeod TC. Caring for student-athletes following a concussion. J Sch Nurs 2009;25(4):270–81.
54. Schneider KJ, Iverson GL, Emery CA, et al. The effects of rest and treatment following sport-related concussion: a systematic review of the literature. Br J Sports Med 2013;47(5):304–7.
55. Collins MW, Lovell MR, Iverson GL, et al. Examining concussion rates and return to play in high school football players wearing newer helmet technology: a three-year prospective cohort study. Neurosurgery 2006;58(2):275–86.
56. Furman JM, Raz Y, Whitney SL. Geriatric vestibulopathy assessment and management. Curr Opin Otolaryngol Head Neck Surg 2010;18(5):386–91.
57. Kapoor N, Ciuffreda KJ. Vision disturbances following traumatic brain injury. Curr Treat Options Neurol 2002;4(4):271–80.
58. Rutner D, Kapoor N, Ciuffreda KJ, et al. Occurrence of ocular disease in traumatic brain injury in a selected sample: a retrospective analysis. Brain Inj 2006; 20(10):1079–86.
59. Stiller-Ostrowski JL. Fourth cranial nerve palsy in a collegiate lacrosse player: a case report. J Athl Train 2010;45(4):407–10.
60. Chan RV, Trobe JD. Spasm of accommodation associated with closed head trauma. J Neuroophthalmol 2002;22(1):15–7.
61. Capo-Aponte JE, Tarbett AK, Urosevich TG, et al. Effectiveness of computerized oculomotor vision screening in a military population: pilot study. J Rehabil Res Dev 2012;49(9):1377–98.
62. Ciuffreda KJ, Rutner D, Kapoor N, et al. Vision therapy for oculomotor dysfunctions in acquired brain injury: a retrospective analysis. Optometry 2008;79(1):18–22.
63. Bhattacharyya N, Baugh RF, Orvidas L, et al. Clinical practice guideline: benign paroxysmal positional vertigo. Otolaryngol Head Neck Surg 2008;139(5 Suppl 4): S47–81.
64. Pavlou M, Bronstein AM, Davies RA. Randomized trial of supervised versus unsupervised optokinetic exercise in persons with peripheral vestibular disorders. Neurorehab & Neu Rep 2013;27:208–18.
65. Furman JM, Marcus DA, Balaban CD. Vestibular migraine: clinical aspects and pathophysiology. Lancet Neurol 2013;12:706–15.
66. Furman JM, Balaban CD, Jacob RG, et al. Migraine-anxiety related dizziness (MARD): a new disorder? J Neurol Neurosurg Psychiatry 2005;76:1–8.
67. Geurts AC, Ribbers GM, Knoop JA, et al. Identification of static and dynamic postural instability following traumatic brain injury. Arch Phys Med Rehabil 1996;77:639–44.
68. Guskiewicz KM. Regaining balance and postural equilibrium. In: Prentice WE, editor. Rehabilitation techniques in sports medicine. 3rd edition. Boston: WCB McGraw-Hill; 1999. p. 107–33.
69. Guskiewicz KM, Riemann BL, Perrin DH, et al. Alternative approaches to the assessment of mild head injury in athletes. Med Sci Sports Exerc 1997;29(7 Suppl):S213–21.

70. Peterson CL, Ferrara MS, Mrazik M, et al. Evaluation of neuropsychological domain scores and postural stability following cerebral concussion in sports. Clin J Sport Med 2003;13(4):230–7.
71. Guskiewicz KM. Postural stability assessment following concussion: one piece of the puzzle. Clin J Sport Med 2001;11(3):182–9.
72. Parker TM, Osternig LR, Lee H, et al. The effect of divided attention on gait stability following concussion. Clin Biomech 2005;20(4):389–95.
73. Catena RD, von Donkelaar P, Chou LS. Cognitive task effects on gait stability following concussion. Exp Brain Res 2007;176(1):23–31.
74. Catena RD, von Donkelaar P, Chou LS. Altered balance control following concussion is better detected with an attention test during gait. Gait Posture 2007;25(3):406–11.
75. Gottshall KR, Hoffer ME. Tracking recovery of vestibular function in individuals with blast-induced head trauma using vestibular-visual-cognitive interaction tests. J Neurol Phys Ther 2010;34(2):94–7.
76. Kozlowski KF, Graham J, Leddy JJ, et al. Exercise intolerance in individuals with postconcussion syndrome. J Athl Train 2013;48(5):627–35.
77. Hillier SL, Hollohan V. Vestibular rehabilitation for unilateral peripheral vestibular dysfunction. Cochrane Database Syst Rev 2007;(4):CD005397.
78. Schneider KJ, Meeuwisse WH, Nettel-Aguirre A, et al. Cervicovestibular rehabilitation in sport-related concussion: a randomised controlled trial. Br J Sports Med 2014;48(17):1294–8.
79. Alsalaheen BA, Mucha A, Morris LO, et al. Vestibular rehabilitation for dizziness and balance disorders after concussion. J Neurol Phys Ther 2010;34(2):87–93.
80. Hoffer ME, Gottshall KR, Moore R, et al. Characterizing and treating dizziness after mild head trauma. Otol Neurotol 2004;25(2):135–8.
81. Scheiman M, Gwiazda J, Li T. Non-surgical interventions for convergence insufficiency. Cochrane Database of Systematic Reviews 2011;CD006768(3).
82. Scheiman M, Cotter S, Kulp MT. Treatment of accommodative dysfunction in children: results from a randomized clinical trial. Optom Vis Sci 2011;88:1343–52.
83. Thiagarajan P, Ciuffreda KJ. Versional eye tracking in mild traumatic brain injury (mTBI): effects of oculomotor training (OMT). Brain Inj 2014;28(7):930–43.
84. Kinnaman KA, Mannix RC, Comstock RD, et al. Management strategies and medication use for treating paediatric patients with concussions. Acta Paediatr 2013;102(9):e424–8.
85. Reddy CC, Collins M, Lovell M, et al. Efficacy of amantadine treatment on symptoms and neurocognitive performance among adolescents following sports-related concussion. J Head Trauma Rehabil 2013;28(4):260–5.
86. Whyte J, Hart T, Vaccaro M, et al. Effects of methylphenidate on attention deficits after traumatic brain injury: a multidimensional, randomized, controlled trial. Am J Phys Med Rehabil 2004;83(6):401–20.
87. Kontos AP, Elbin RJ, Lau B, et al. Posttraumatic migraine as a predictor of recovery and cognitive impairment after sport-related concussion. Am J Sports Med 2013;41(7):1497–504.
88. Petraglia AL, Maroon JC, Bailes JE. From the field of play to the field of combat: a review of the pharmacological management of concussion. Neurosurgery 2012;70(6):1520–33 [discussion: 1533].
89. Meehan WP. Medical therapies for concussion. Clin Sports Med 2011;30(1):115–24.
90. Pavlou M, Davies RA, Bronstein AM. The assessment of increased sensitivity to visual stimuli in patients with chronic dizziness. J Vestib Res 2006;16(4–5):223–31.

91. Guskiewicz KM, Ross SE, Marshall SW. Postural stability and neuropsychological deficits after concussion in collegiate athletes. J Athl Train 2001;36(3):263–73.

92. Norre ME. Cervical vertigo. Diagnostic and semiological problem with special emphasis upon "cervical nystagmus". Acta Otorhinolaryngol Belg 1987;41(3): 436–52.

93. Kristjansson E, Treleaven J. Sensorimotor function and dizziness in neck pain: implications for assessment and management. J Orthop Sports Phys Ther 2009; 39(5):364–77.

94. Leddy JJ, Kozlowski K, Fung M, et al. Regulatory and autoregulatory physiological dysfunction as a primary characteristic of post concussion syndrome: implications for treatment. NeuroRehabilitation 2007;22(3):199–205.

Knowing the Speed Limit

Weighing the Benefits and Risks of Rehabilitation Progression After Arthroscopic Rotator Cuff Repair

Charles A. Thigpen, PT, PhD, ATC[a,b,*],
Michael A. Shaffer, MSPT, OCS, ATC[c], Michael J. Kissenberth, MD[d]

KEYWORDS

- Rotator cuff repair • Range of motion • Outcomes • Rehabilitation

KEY POINTS

- The "speed limit" for rehabilitation after rotator cuff repair is based on patient-centric factors, including tear chronicity, tissue quality, the ability to meet staged goals, and tolerance to rehabilitation stresses.
- Structural failure (nonhealing or retear) after rotator cuff repair is not uncommon (25%–60%), but is not consistently associated with worse functional outcomes.
- To provide the best environment for healing, immobilization and limited passive range of motion (ROM) should be considered during the first 6 weeks after rotator cuff repair.
- Postoperative stiffness for >6 months is not common (3%–10%), but at-risk individuals benefit from additional focus on their passive ROM earlier in the immediate postoperative period.
- Gains in ROM in accelerated programs result in moderate gains in forward elevation and external rotation ROM at 6 months, which are not likely impactful on patient function.

INTRODUCTION

Rotator cuff repairs are becoming increasingly common resulting in direct medical costs exceeding $7 billion per year in the United States.[1–4] At present, the number of rotator cuff repairs exceeds 450,000 surgeries per year with more than 95% being performed arthroscopically,[5] Studies consistently demonstrate good to excellent patient outcomes after rotator cuff repair, independent of rotator cuff integrity, at 2-year follow

[a] Proaxis Therapy, 200 Patewood Drive, Suite 150 C, Greenville, SC, USA; [b] Center for Rehabilitation and Reconstruction Sciences, Greenville, SC, USA; [c] Department of Rehabilitation Therapies, University of Iowa Hospitals and Clinics, Iowa City, IA, USA; [d] Department of Orthopedics, Steadman-Hawkins Clinics of the Carolinas, Greenville Health System, Greenville, SC, USA
* Corresponding author. Proaxis Therapy, 200 Patewood Drive, Suite 150 C, Greenville, SC.
E-mail address: chuck.thigpen@proaxistherapy.com

Clin Sports Med 34 (2015) 233–246
http://dx.doi.org/10.1016/j.csm.2014.12.007
0278-5919/15/$ – see front matter © 2015 Elsevier Inc. All rights reserved.

up.[6–16] These studies typically include a broadly described supervised rehabilitation protocol, which suggests that supervised therapy is an important component in the ideal treatment of rotator cuff tears.[17] Recently, a number of randomized trials, systematic reviews, and meta-analyses have examined the duration of immobilization and the initiation of range of motion (ROM) progression. Taken together, these papers suggest a period of immobilization (usually 6 weeks) and protected early ROM, followed by a systematic rehabilitation progression of active ROM, strengthening, and functional activities. This approach of protected, passive ROM concurrent with or after a period of immobilization results in similar outcomes with higher rates of structural healing compared with an approach of immediate ROM without limits.

However, these randomized, controlled trials primarily address patients with tears that are less than 3 cm, have good tissue quality, and do not have many of the factors that potentially influence functional and structural outcomes after rotator cuff repair. Functional and structural outcomes are negatively influenced by advanced age of the individual, activity level of the patient, duration of symptoms, extent of the tear, location of the tear, the number of tendons involved, rotator cuff tissue quality, atrophy of muscles, and associated shoulder pathology.[18–21] Given that these factors are not uncommon in some patients undergoing rotator cuff repair, it is confusing as to how the results of the randomized, controlled trials should be applied across the spectrum of patients after rotator cuff repair. Thus, the purpose of this paper was to link clinical rehabilitation practice with the literature and describe the factors that, in our opinion, should be considered when determining the appropriate "speed limit" of a patient-centered postoperative rehabilitation plan after rotator cuff repair.

THE CONTROVERSY

The struggle when to initiate and progress patients after rotator cuff repair is anchored by 2 seemingly opposing clinical concerns: prevention of postoperative stiffness and maintenance of structural integrity. These concerns frame the crux of the decisions when determining the rate of progression after rotator cuff repair.

1. *Structural integrity:* Arthroscopic rotator cuff repairs provide reliable satisfactory clinical outcomes despite wide ranges of structural healing from 16% to 94%.[5,8,12,22,23] The results do not seem to independently drive intermediate (1–2 years) functional outcome.[6–16]
2. *Postoperative stiffness:* Initiation of immediate (beginning the day after surgery) motion with few or no limits is thought to prevent stiffness considered to be the result of increased adhesions and scar tissue formation in the subdeltoid and subacromial spaces.[24–26] This activity is usually followed by an accelerated progression to active ROM, and resistive and functional activities, which result in an earlier return to activities.[27]

The rehabilitation clinician must weigh the benefits of early initiation (<4–6 weeks) of ROM and a faster progression through the phases of rehabilitation against the increased risks of structural failure. This decision is made in the context of the risk factors for failure as well as the risk factors for stiffness, including calcific tendonitis, adhesive capsulitis, partial articular surface tendon avulsion, type of rotator cuff repair, concomitant labral repair, or an acute, single-tendon cuff repair.[18–21]

Injury History and Prior Treatment

When planning rehabilitation after rotator cuff repair, it is important to consider the suspected underlying mechanisms of how the rotator cuff ruptured. Compressive and shear forces at the bursal and articular side of the tendon are thought to result in degenerative intratendinous partial tears.[28–31] These microtears proliferate over time, creating tension overloads in the remaining tendon, exacerbating force concentration in the remaining tendon tissue, which leads to complete full-thickness failure.[32] The majority of rotator cuff tears are understood to be complete tendon failure from this cumulative attrition (atraumatic, chronic tear) or from a sudden force that exceeds the structural integrity of the already degenerated tissue (acute traumatic tear on chronic tissue). The final mechanism is an acute tear from a larger force (ie, dislocation) in previously healthy tissue. Except in cases of acute tears, the repaired rotator cuff is not a normal tendon and is thought to be a contributing mechanism to the structural failure after repair. This circumstance means the healing environment is often less than ideal and makes healing more tenuous. Thus, a more conservative rate of rehabilitation is prudent in the postoperative condition and more so for those patients in whom healing is even more of a concern.

The history of the tear provides important prognosis and postoperative planning considerations. Atraumatic tears with no clear onset mechanism often respond well to nonoperative rehabilitation.[17,33–35] In contrast, acute tears with rapid onset of weakness are repaired early (within 2–3 months).[36,37] Although there seems to be a role for a trial of nonoperative management of rotator cuff tears, increased postoperative strength and decreased pain have been correlated with early surgical repair.[38–40] Typically, those cases with smaller tears and a shorter duration of symptoms before repair have had better clinical outcomes.[39,41] Understanding the patient's response to nonoperative management and their unresolved complaint that resulted in their choice to undergo surgery can aid in planning their postoperative course. Conversely, identifying which impairments responded to preoperative treatment allows for a more focused postoperative rehabilitation plan.

Rotator Cuff Repair Integrity

The integrity of the rotator cuff repair must be considered when determining the postoperative rehabilitation plan. The initial integrity of the repair is a combined result of the tissue quality of the rotator cuff tendon, the operative technique, and the surgical materials used.[42–47] For example, a healthy tendon with a double row repair[48] might initiate motion earlier and progress to active ROM and resistive exercises faster compared with an a thinner, more degenerative tendon with a medialized single row repair.[49,50] The double row repair is a solid construct, which is less likely to fail from gradual application of stress, whereas the single row in a more degenerative setting is at risk for failure. The starting point is earlier and the speed limit is faster for the former. However, even the most ideal setting, the healed rotator cuff does not recover to normal biomechanical properties in terms of elasticity and maximum strength until well after 6 months postoperatively.[42,45,51] This gradual improvement suggests that, for the first 6 months, significant activity modifications and limitations should be considered for nearly all patients. **Table 1** provides a protocol to facilitate communication between the surgeon and therapist. It is divided into protocols for tears that are less than 3 cm and greater than 3 cm[52,53] (as measured in the coronal plane), with longer immobilization and delayed initiation of passive ROM for the large and massive rotator cuff tears. Although the size of the tear dictates the duration of immobilization, the rate of the rehabilitation progression is determined by associated factors of tissue quality and healing. For the purposes of simplicity, the rate of progression was held constant between the 2 tear sizes presented in **Table 1**. That is, the decisions a rehabilitation clinician makes that alter the rehabilitation progression and ultimately

Table 1
Proaxis Therapy: Steadman Hawkins Clinics of the Carolinas rotator cuff protocol

Stage	<3 cm in Coronal Plane	>3 cm in Coronal Plane

Immobilization	Sling with pillow for weeks 0–3
	Regular sling (remove pillow) for
	  weeks 3–6
		Sling with pillow for weeks 0–4
		Regular sling (remove pillow) for
		  weeks 4–8

Phase 0 (quiet)	**Weeks 0–1:**
	Quiet in sling with elbow/wrist/hand
	Begin active scapular retraction/
	  protraction exercises with
	  therapist cueing
		Weeks 0–4:
		Quiet in sling with elbow/wrist/hand
		Begin active scapular retraction/
		  protraction exercises with
		  therapist cueing

Phase 1 (passive)	Pendulums to begin
	Weeks 2–6:
	Supine external rotation: 0°–30°
	  beginning at 2 wk with
	  progression to full PROM by 6 wk
	Supine forward elevation: 0°–90°
	  beginning at 2 wk with
	  progression to full PROM by 6 wk
	Progress to upright as tolerated with
	  ER and FE
		Pendulums to begin
		Weeks 5–8:
		Supine external rotation: 0°–30°
		  beginning at 5 wk with
		  progression to full PROM by 8 wk
		Supine forward elevation: 0°–90°
		  beginning at 5 wk with
		  progression to full PROM by 8 wk
		Progress to upright as tolerated with
		  ER and FE

Phase 2 (active)	Pendulums to warm-up
	AROM with terminal stretch
	Weeks 7–9:
	Supine external rotation – after 6 wk
	  progress gradually to full
	Supine forward elevation – after
	  6 wk; progress gradually to full
	Begin active biceps
	Internal rotation—full (begin
	  behind the back)
	Begin AROM in supine and progress
	  to upright
		Pendulums to warm-up
		AROM with terminal stretch
		Weeks 9–12:
		Supine external rotation – after 8 wk
		  progress gradually to full
		Supine forward elevation – after
		  8 wk; progress gradually to full
		Begin active biceps
		Internal rotation—full (begin
		  behind the back)
		Begin AROM in supine and progress
		  to upright

Phase 3 (resisted)	**Week 10:** External and internal rotation Standing forward punch Seated rows Shoulder shrugs and biceps curls	**Week 13:** External and internal rotation Standing forward punch Seated rows Shoulder shrugs and biceps curls

Weight training	**Week 12:**
	Keep hands within eyesight, keep
	  elbows bent, no long lever arms
	Minimize overhead activities (below
	  shoulder)
	No military press, pull-down behind
	  head, or wide grip bench
		Week 16:
		Keep hands within eyesight, keep
		  elbows bent, no long lever arms
		Minimize overhead activities (below
		  shoulder)
		No military press, pull-down behind
		  head, or wide grip bench

Initiation of
  interval sports
  programs
	Golf: 3–4 mo
	Tennis: 5–6 mo
	Ski: 5–6 mo
		Golf: 5–6 mo
		Tennis: 7–8 mo
		Ski: 7–8 mo

Immediate start to physical therapy for education, home exercise compliance postoperative day 1–3. Gradual progression of activities and exercises per protocol after the approximate ROM targets for each phase.

Abbreviations: AROM, active range of motion; ER, external rotation; FE, forward elevation; PROM, passive range of motion; ROM, range of motion.

help to determine the speed limit of rehabilitation are explained elsewhere in this article, rather than in the more broad categories that are delineated in **Table 1**.

The delay in the initiation of ROM for tears greater than 3 cm is because many larger tears also have associated muscle atrophy and fatty infiltration. Both factors are strongly associated with reparability and integrity with reports of structural failure (nonhealing or retearing) from 25% to 93%.[54–60] This may explain why larger tears have been shown to fail earlier than smaller tears[61,62] and why larger tears are more at risk for structural failure with more aggressive rehabilitation timelines in randomized, controlled trials.[63] Based on the available clinical evidence, it seems that larger tears should be cautiously approached during the first 12 weeks postoperatively. However, no studies that we are aware of have specifically examined the effects of atrophy or fatty infiltration on postoperative functional outcomes independent of structural failure. In sum, clinicians should consider the repair and tissue integrity and appropriately adjust the rate of progression, the specific therapeutic interventions, and the course of an individual's postoperative rehabilitation plan.

Tendon Healing

The primary risk for structural failure after arthroscopic rotator cuff repair is the tendon itself, because modern suture anchor/suture constructs are not apt to fail.[45,64] Structural healing of the rotator cuff tendon only occurs with surgical, tension-free repair of the rotator cuff tendon back to its footprint on the tuberosity.[44,65] Healing principally occurs from the bone to the tendon—beginning around 21 to 28 days after repair—for the synthesis of new tissue and the remodeling of scar tissue based on imposed loads. Although tensile strength improves dramatically after 12 weeks, animal studies consistently demonstrate gapping of repaired defects and inadequate mechanical properties until after 6 months.[18,43,66,67] Thus, careful consideration of the influence of motion on the healing rotator cuff is important. Contrary to the traditional view that early motion decreases adhesions and promotes tissue elongation,[68] recent evidence suggests that early motion actually increases collagen formation within the subacromial space.[69–73] This strategy results in a stiffer construct initially of unorganized type III collagen, but a weaker tendon when compared with tendons that were completely immobilized. Additionally, immobilized tendons showed decreased motion at 4 weeks, but these deficits were resolved by 8 weeks postoperatively. Not only did the joint motion return, but tendons, which were loaded later displayed more type I collagen, which resulted in a more organized and stronger construct when compared with the early motion group.[74] In sum, this basic science work suggests that immobilization followed by gradual progression of loading and ROM actually facilitates a stronger tendon interface after rotator cuff repair than does an approach of immediate motion.

The struggle with incorporating this evidence into clinical practice is that recent randomized, controlled trials, systematic reviews, and meta-analyses show equal patient reported outcomes at 1 to 2 years of follow-up.[75–81] However, the randomized, controlled trials were powered to evaluate patient function, not structural healing rates. What is not clear is the long-term impact of structural healing on patient outcomes. Thus, considering the timing of the structural failure in the context of tear size may help to guide clinical practice. Ninety-eight percent of patients presented with structural failure (nonhealing or retear) within the first 6 months after repair regardless of tear size.[61,62] However, among the larger tears (>4 cm) 78% failed within the first 3 months,[45] whereas failure of smaller tears (<4 cm) occurred more evenly over the first 6 months.[10] These results agree with the recent meta-analysis, which showed large, massive tears were nearly at 2 times greater risk for structural failure in studies that used an initiation of early motion. Structural failure is associated with strength deficits. Larger tears show concurrent decreased health-related quality of life.[82] The combination, of basic science and clinical studies, suggests that initial immobilization and protected ROM for 4 to 6 weeks result in similar patient outcomes at 1 to 2 years, with improved healing rates and without residual postoperative stiffness compared with the early, unprotected ROM approach.[18,77,81,83,84] However, older patients (>65), with larger tears (>4 cm), with poor tissue quality, greater tendon retraction, or tears not restored to the footprint in a tension-free manner should undergo longer immobilization and delay of ROM exercises for 8 to 12 weeks.[82,85–89] In addition to a more deliberate progression through rehabilitation phases, that is, a slower speed limit, the prolonged immobilization period for these patients is considered to provide the best opportunity for the rotator cuff repair to heal, and providing the best chance for long-term outcomes.

Postoperative Stiffness

The incidence of postoperative shoulder stiffness after arthroscopic rotator cuff repair is relatively low (3%–10%), and is reported to resolve usually with therapy or watchful waiting within the first year after surgery.[18,27,90–92] Intermediate postoperative stiffness (3–6 months) associated with an initial immobilization period and/or protected motion phase is reported (5%–23%), and on average results in a 15° deficit in forward elevation and 7° in neutral, external rotation. These limitations in ROM are not likely to result in significant alterations in patient function and are consistently resolved by 1 year.

Recalcitrant postoperative stiffness seems to be uncommon after rotator cuff repair, but there are several factors associated with persistent ROM deficits, including calcific tendonitis, adhesive capsulitis, partial articular surface tendon avulsion, type of rotator cuff repair, concomitant labral repair, or an acute, single-tendon cuff repair.[18–21] Even in patients at risk for postoperative stiffness, a simple addition of unweighted exercise for forward elevation equalized the risk of stiffness with rotator cuff repair without those factors (**Fig. 1**A, B).[20] Given the relatively minimal amounts of supraspinatus activity with these exercises,[93,94] it would seem that patients at risk for stiffness benefit from early motion after rotator cuff repair.

PROGRESSION BETWEEN PHASES AND MANAGEMENT OF COMPLICATIONS

Impairments, such as pain, ROM, and strength, are expected to improve every 1 to 2 weeks after rotator cuff repair; patient-rated outcome measures show improvement every 2 to 4 weeks. A combination of patient-rated and clinician-measured outcomes should be used to establish rehabilitation priorities and guide the rate of progression through the rehabilitation process. We recommend the use of the Western Ontario Rotator Cuff Index or the Pennsylvania Shoulder Score or American Shoulder and Elbow Surgeon form, patient-rated section, for measuring patient-rated outcomes.[95–99] The key clinical impairments include pain at rest, forward elevation ROM, and external rotation ROM with the arm by the side. Later in the rehabilitation process, rotator cuff strength with the arm the side and the ability to raise the hand overhead with appropriate scapulohumeral rhythm can also be used as gauges of rehabilitation progress. Although we acknowledge that there is much other impairment that may impact shoulder function, these impairments provide simple measures to examine overall shoulder function. Although progression from phase to phase is based on achievement of each phase's milestones, when the expected milestones are not achieved, the rehabilitation clinician should collaborate with the referring surgeon on any

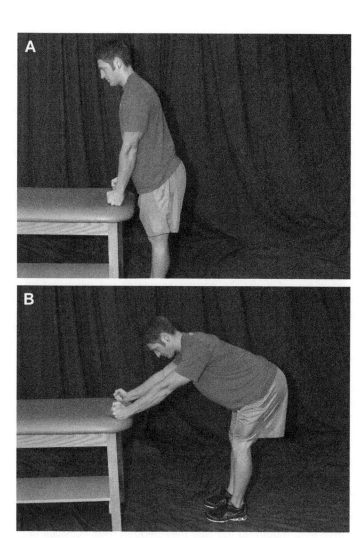

Fig. 1. Patient rests hands on counter/table to unweight the arm then "walks back" to prescribed range of motion target.

significant changes to rehabilitation goals. Signs and symptoms suggesting poor tolerance of the rehabilitation progression include the following.

- Complaints pain at rest/night (>6/10) for phases 0 and 1, (>4/10) for phase 2, and (>2/10) after phase 3.
- Greater than 20° lag in ROM goals per stage.
- Inability to demonstrate active elevation or gross loss of strength after 8 to 12 weeks.

When these signs of poor tolerance to rehabilitation are present, patient education and an adjusted treatment plan is most often all that is necessary get the patient "back on track." For instance, early in the rehabilitation process many patients experience discomfort when they perform their initial ROM exercises. Most often either the patients are performing their exercises beyond the desired level of "stretch" and/or are not keeping their involved limb relaxed during the ROM exercises. In this situation, the rehabilitation clinician needs to clarify the goals of the initial ROM work (to guard against developing postoperative stiffness rather than truly restore preoperative ROM) and ensure that the patient is performing the exercises with the correct amount of support of the involved limb.

Stiffness, or the inability to achieve staged ROM goals, should be carefully evaluated and likely warrants closely supervised rehabilitation. The key clinical decision when ROM is lagging is whether the deficits are primarily owing to pain or true restriction of joint mobility. When pain predominates, the rehabilitation clinician may need to slow the speed of the rehabilitation progression and advise the patient to use their sling, undergo cryotherapy, and perform anti-inflammatory modalities until resting pain is again controlled. Once resting pain is controlled, then gentle passive ROM/active assistive ROM exercises can be restarted. Conversely, if pain is controlled, but the end feel is "tight," which is rare except in a few particular situations (partial thickness tears, calcific tendonitis, adhesive capsulitis), then increasing the number of supervised rehabilitation visits per week or the frequency at which the home exercise program is performed is the most prudent response. Increasing the intensity of the stretching is almost never the correct approach; the rehabilitation clinician is reminded that healing after rotator cuff repair is tenuous and ROM deficits are generally short lived.

Only when the patient has achieved the ROM goals and has their pain well-controlled are they ready to progress to the next phase of rehabilitation. A patient whose pain is well-controlled because they are not regularly performing their ROM exercises or a patient who is achieving the staged ROM goals, but is only able to do so with considerable pain, is not ready to progress. In either of these scenarios, the rate of progression—the speed limit of rehabilitation—must be slowed.

Although successfully initiating ROM work is a common difficulty of rehabilitation, it is not the only difficult progression. Occasionally, patients will start to experience increased pain when active ROM or resistance exercises are begun. Chronologically, this progression to "strengthening"-type exercises shortly follows a time when patients have discontinued use of their slings and have returned to many activities of daily living. Any one of these changes—discontinuing use of their sling, resuming activities of daily living, or starting a phase of exercises that places more stress on the healing tendon—may increase a patient's pain. Luckily, teaching a patient about supporting their arm, modifying the way they perform their activities of daily living, or emphasizing pain relief and passive ROM exercises while deemphasizing "strengthening" usually gets patients back on track. Again, it is imperative that the rehabilitation specialist recognize the warning signs that the patient is not tolerating the current speed of the rehabilitation process and slow the rate of progress.

When patients present with an inability to regain active elevation or a persistent inability to regain strength, the surgeon should be informed as soon as possible. The rehabilitation clinician must ensure that the patient has appropriate passive forward elevation. If the patient has adequate passive elevation, the patient should perform a progressive active elevation program beginning in supine and gradually increasing the influence of gravity. This progression is particularly helpful if the patient has an intact rotator cuff, but is having difficulty regaining control of the muscle power in elevated positions. Finally, focus on rotator cuff function, in a shortened lever arm position, that is, elbow bent, is also helpful to maximize active elevation.

During the rehabilitation process, any time difficulty is encountered and the patient is not making the expected gains, it is crucial that the surgeon and therapist work together to adjust the treatment plan, and clarify the expected outcomes/goals as well as the speed limit for the rehabilitation progression.

SUMMARY

Immobilization, initiation of ROM, progression of exercises, and activities of daily living after rotator cuff repair are common challenges to the patient, surgeon, and rehabilitation professional after rotator cuff repair. Many factors influence the structural integrity of the repair and the ultimate patient outcome. Considering these factors and communicating this information among the surgeon, therapist, and patient allow a patient-centered rehabilitation plan. Individually adjusting the speed of rehabilitation for the patient's age and expectations, as well as the rotator cuff tear size, tissue quality and repair integrity, produce a more comprehensive path. An initial period of immobilization based on these factors, combined with a focus on controlled, protected passive ROM and then a gradual loading beyond 12 weeks, is recommended based on the best available basic science and clinical studies to date. Difficulties with achieving staged goals necessitate a modification of the rehabilitation plan and perhaps an alteration of the speed limit of the rehabilitation process.

REFERENCES

1. Mall NA, Kim HM, Keener JD, et al. Symptomatic progression of asymptomatic rotator cuff tears: a prospective study of clinical and sonographic variables. J Bone Joint Surg Am 2010;92(16):2623–33.
2. Milgrom C, Schaffler M, Gilbert S, et al. Rotator-cuff changes in asymptomatic adults. The effect of age, hand dominance and gender. J Bone Joint Surg Br 1995;77(2):296–8.
3. Reilly P, Macleod I, Macfarlane R, et al. Dead men and radiologists don't lie: a review of cadaveric and radiological studies of rotator cuff tear prevalence. Ann R Coll Surg Engl 2006;88(2):116–21.
4. Yamamoto A, Takagishi K, Osawa T, et al. Prevalence and risk factors of a rotator cuff tear in the general population. J Shoulder Elbow Surg 2010;19(1):116–20.
5. Cole BJ, McCarty LP 3rd, Kang RW, et al. Arthroscopic rotator cuff repair: prospective functional outcome and repair integrity at minimum 2-year follow-up. J Shoulder Elbow Surg 2007;16(5):579–85.
6. Bishop J, Klepps S, Lo IK, et al. Cuff integrity after arthroscopic versus open rotator cuff repair: a prospective study. J Shoulder Elbow Surg 2006;15(3):290–9.
7. Charousset C, Grimberg J, Duranthon LD, et al. The time for functional recovery after arthroscopic rotator cuff repair: correlation with tendon healing controlled by computed tomography arthrography. Arthroscopy 2008;24(1):25–33.
8. DeFranco MJ, Bershadsky B, Ciccone J, et al. Functional outcome of arthroscopic rotator cuff repairs: a correlation of anatomic and clinical results. J Shoulder Elbow Surg 2007;16(6):759–65.
9. Gerber C, Fuchs B, Hodler J, et al. The results of repair of massive tears of the rotator cuff. J Bone Joint Surg Am 2000;82(4):505–15.
10. Gerber C, Schneeberger AG, Beck M, et al. Mechanical strength of repairs of the rotator cuff. J Bone Joint Surg Br 1994;76(3):371–80.
11. Goutallier D, Postel JM, Bernageau J, et al. Fatty muscle degeneration in cuff ruptures. Pre- and postoperative evaluation by CT scan. Clin Orthop Relat Res 1994;(304):78–83.

12. Harryman DT 2nd, Mack LA, Wang KY, et al. Repairs of the rotator cuff. Correlation of functional results with integrity of the cuff. J Bone Joint Surg Am 1991;73: 982–9.

13. Jost B, Pfirrmann CW, Gerber C, et al. Clinical outcome after structural failure of rotator cuff repairs. J Bone Joint Surg Am 2000;82(3):304–14.

14. Liu SH, Baker CL. Arthroscopically assisted rotator cuff repair: correlation of functional results with integrity of the cuff. Arthroscopy 1994;10(1):54–60.

15. Severud EL, Ruotolo C, Abbott DD, et al. All-arthroscopic versus mini-open rotator cuff repair: A long-term retrospective outcome comparison. Arthroscopy 2003; 19(3):234–8.

16. Thomazeau H, Boukobza E, Morcet N, et al. Prediction of rotator cuff repair results by magnetic resonance imaging. Clin Orthop Relat Res 1997;(344): 275–83.

17. Kuhn JE, Dunn WR, Sanders R, et al. Effectiveness of physical therapy in treating atraumatic full-thickness rotator cuff tears: a multicenter prospective cohort study. J Shoulder Elbow Surg 2013;22:1371–9.

18. Denard PJ, Ladermann A, Burkhart SS. Prevention and management of stiffness after arthroscopic rotator cuff repair: systematic review and implications for rotator cuff healing. Arthroscopy 2011;27(6):842–8.

19. Huberty DP, Schoolfield JD, Brady PC, et al. Incidence and treatment of postoperative stiffness following arthroscopic rotator cuff repair. Arthroscopy 2009;25(8): 880–90.

20. Koo SS, Parsley BK, Burkhart SS, et al. Reduction of postoperative stiffness after arthroscopic rotator cuff repair: results of a customized physical therapy regimen based on risk factors for stiffness. Arthroscopy 2011;27(2):155–60.

21. Oh JH, Kim SH, Lee HK, et al. Moderate preoperative shoulder stiffness does not alter the clinical outcome of rotator cuff repair with arthroscopic release and manipulation. Arthroscopy 2008;24(9):983–91.

22. Galatz LM, Ball CM, Teefey SA, et al. The outcome and repair integrity of completely arthroscopically repaired large and massive rotator cuff tears. J Bone Joint Surg Am 2004;86-A(2):219–24.

23. Meyer M, Klouche S, Rousselin B, et al. Does arthroscopic rotator cuff repair actually heal? Anatomic evaluation with magnetic resonance arthrography at minimum 2 years follow-up. J Shoulder Elbow Surg 2012;21:531–6.

24. Lastayo PC, Wright T, Jaffe R, et al. Continuous passive motion after repair of the rotator cuff. A prospective outcome study. J Bone Joint Surg Am 1998;80(7):1002–11.

25. Norberg FB, Field LD, Savoie FH 3rd, et al. Repair of the rotator cuff. Mini-open and arthroscopic repairs. Clin Sports Med 2000;19(1):77–99.

26. Raab MG, Rzeszutko D, O'Connor W, et al. Early results of continuous passive motion after rotator cuff repair: a prospective, randomized, blinded, controlled study. Am J Orthop (Belle Mead NJ) 1996;25(3):214–20.

27. Parsons BO, Gruson KI, Chen DD, et al. Does slower rehabilitation after arthroscopic rotator cuff repair lead to long-term stiffness? J Shoulder Elbow Surg 2010;19(7):1034–9.

28. Burkhart SS. Arthroscopic treatment of massive rotator cuff tears. Clinical results and biomechanical rationale. Clin Orthop Relat Res 1991;(267):45–56.

29. Burkhart SS. Biomechanics of rotator cuff repair: converting the ritual to a science. Instr Course Lect 1998;47:43–50.

30. Reilly P, Amis AA, Wallace AL, et al. Mechanical factors in the initiation and propagation of tears of the rotator cuff. Quantification of strains of the supraspinatus tendon in vitro. J Bone Joint Surg Br 2003;85(4):594–9.

31. Seitz AL, McClure PW, Finucane S, et al. Mechanisms of rotator cuff tendinopathy: intrinsic, extrinsic, or both? Clin Biomech (Bristol, Avon) 2011;26(1):1–12.
32. Soslowsky LJ, Thomopoulos S, Esmail A, et al. Rotator cuff tendinosis in an animal model: role of extrinsic and overuse factors. Ann Biomed Eng 2002;30(8): 1057–63.
33. Brophy RH, Dunn WR, Kuhn JE. Shoulder activity level is not associated with the severity of symptomatic, atraumatic rotator cuff tears in patients electing nonoperative treatment. Am J Sports Med 2014;42(5):1150–4.
34. Dunn WR, Kuhn JE, Sanders R, et al. Symptoms of pain do not correlate with rotator cuff tear severity: a cross-sectional study of 393 patients with a symptomatic atraumatic full-thickness rotator cuff tear. J Bone Joint Surg Am 2014;96(10): 793–800.
35. Unruh KP, Kuhn JE, Sanders R, et al. The duration of symptoms does not correlate with rotator cuff tear severity or other patient-related features: a cross-sectional study of patients with atraumatic, full-thickness rotator cuff tears. J Shoulder Elbow Surg 2014;23(7):1052–8.
36. Butler BR, Byrne AN, Higgins LD, et al. Results of the repair of acute rotator cuff tears is not influenced by tear retraction. Int J Shoulder Surg 2013;7(3):91–9.
37. Shields E, Mirabelli M, Amsdell S, et al. Functional and imaging outcomes of arthroscopic simultaneous rotator cuff repair and bankart repair after shoulder dislocations. Am J Sports Med 2014;42:2614–20.
38. Bassett RW, Cofield RH. Acute tears of the rotator cuff. The timing of surgical repair. Clin Orthop Relat Res 1983;(175):18–24.
39. Bjorkenheim JM, Paavolainen P, Ahovuo J, et al. Surgical repair of the rotator cuff and surrounding tissues. Factors influencing the results. Clin Orthop Relat Res 1988;(236):148–53.
40. Cofield RH, Parvizi J, Hoffmeyer PJ, et al. Surgical repair of chronic rotator cuff tears. A prospective long-term study. J Bone Joint Surg Am 2001;83-A(1): 71–7.
41. Hawkins RJ, Misamore GW, Hobeika PE. Surgery for full-thickness rotator-cuff tears. J Bone Joint Surg Am 1985;67(9):1349–55.
42. Burkhart SS, Johnson TC, Wirth MA, et al. Cyclic loading of transosseous rotator cuff repairs: tension overload as a possible cause of failure. Arthroscopy 1997; 13(2):172–6.
43. Carpenter JE, Thomopoulos S, Flanagan CL, et al. Rotator cuff defect healing: a biomechanical and histologic analysis in an animal model. J Shoulder Elbow Surg 1998;7(6):599–605.
44. Galatz LM, Rothermich SY, Zaegel M, et al. Delayed repair of tendon to bone injuries leads to decreased biomechanical properties and bone loss. J Orthop Res 2005;23(6):1441–7.
45. Gerber C, Schneeberger AG, Beck M, et al. Mechanical strength of repairs of the rotator cuff. J Bone Joint Surg Br 1994;76(3):371–80.
46. Killian ML, Cavinatto L, Galatz LM, et al. The role of mechanobiology in tendon healing. J Shoulder Elbow Surg 2012;21(2):228–37.
47. Thomopoulos S, Williams GR, Soslowsky LJ. Tendon to bone healing: differences in biomechanical, structural, and compositional properties due to a range of activity levels. J Biomech Eng 2003;125(1):106–13.
48. Saridakis P, Jones G. Outcomes of single-row and double-row arthroscopic rotator cuff repair: a systematic review. J Bone Joint Surg 2010;92(3):732–42.
49. Kim KC, Shin HD, Kim BK, et al. Changes in tendon length with increasing rotator cuff tear size. Knee Surg Sports Traumatol Arthrosc 2012;20(6):1022–6.

50. Tashjian RZ, Hung M, Burks RT, et al. Influence of preoperative musculotendinous junction position on rotator cuff healing using single-row technique. Arthroscopy 2013;29(11):1748–54.
51. Guelich D, Mundanthanam GJ, Govea C, et al. Effects of rehabilitation on cuff integrity and range of motion following arthroscopic cuff repair. Paper presented at AAOS Annual Meeting. 2007.
52. Kuhn JE, Dunn WR, Ma B, et al. Interobserver agreement in the classification of rotator cuff tears. Am J Sports Med 2007;35(3):437–41.
53. Spencer EE Jr, Dunn WR, Wright RW, et al. Interobserver agreement in the classification of rotator cuff tears using magnetic resonance imaging. Am J Sports Med 2008;36(1):99–103.
54. Demirors H, Circi E, Akgun RC, et al. Correlations of isokinetic measurements with tendon healing following open repair of rotator cuff tears. Int Orthop 2009;34:531–6.
55. Gerber C, Schneeberger AG, Hoppeler H, et al. Correlation of atrophy and fatty infiltration on strength and integrity of rotator cuff repairs: a study in thirteen patients. J Shoulder Elbow Surg 2007;16(6):691–6.
56. Jost B, Zumstein M, Pfirrmann CW, et al. Long-term outcome after structural failure of rotator cuff repairs. J Bone Joint Surg Am 2006;88(3):472–9.
57. Rulewicz GJ, Beaty S, Hawkins RJ, et al. Supraspinatus atrophy as a predictor of rotator cuff tear size: an MRI study utilizing the tangent sign. J Shoulder Elbow Surg 2013;22(6):e6–10.
58. Gladstone JN, Bishop JY, Lo IK, et al. Fatty infiltration and atrophy of the rotator cuff do not improve after rotator cuff repair and correlate with poor functional outcome. Am J Sports Med 2007;35(5):719–28.
59. Harris JD, Pedroza A, Jones GL. Predictors of pain and function in patients with symptomatic, atraumatic full-thickness rotator cuff tears: a time-zero analysis of a prospective patient cohort enrolled in a structured physical therapy program. Am J Sports Med 2012;40(2):359–66.
60. Thomazeau H, Boukobza E, Morcet N, et al. Prediction of rotator cuff repair results by magnetic resonance imaging. Clin Orthop Relat Res 1997;(344):275–83.
61. Iannotti JP, Deutsch A, Green A, et al. Time to failure after rotator cuff repair: a prospective imaging study. J Bone Joint Surg Am 2013;95(11):965–71.
62. Miller BS, Downie BK, Kohen RB, et al. When do rotator cuff repairs fail? Serial ultrasound examination after arthroscopic repair of large and massive rotator cuff tears. Am J Sports Med 2011;39(10):2064–70.
63. Chang KV, Hung CY, Han DS, et al. Early versus delayed passive range of motion exercise for arthroscopic rotator cuff repair: a meta-analysis of randomized controlled trials. Am J Sports Med 2014. [Epub ahead of print].
64. Bicknell RT, Harwood C, Ferreira L, et al. Cyclic loading of rotator cuff repairs: an in vitro biomechanical comparison of bioabsorbable tacks with transosseous sutures. Arthroscopy 2005;21(7):875–80.
65. Galatz LM, Charlton N, Das R, et al. Complete removal of load is detrimental to rotator cuff healing. J Shoulder Elbow Surg 2009;18(5):669–75.
66. Keener JD, Wei AS, Kim HM, et al. Revision arthroscopic rotator cuff repair: repair integrity and clinical outcome. J Bone Joint Surg Am 2010;92(3):590–8.
67. Kim HM, Dahiya N, Teefey SA, et al. Relationship of tear size and location to fatty degeneration of the rotator cuff. J Bone Joint Surg Am 2010;92(4):829–39.
68. Lee TQ. Current biomechanical concepts for rotator cuff repair. Clin Orthop Surg 2013;5(2):89–97.
69. Peltz CD, Dourte LM, Kuntz AF, et al. The effect of postoperative passive motion on rotator cuff healing in a rat model. J Bone Joint Surg Am 2009;91(10):2421–9.

70. Peltz CD, Sarver JJ, Dourte LM, et al. Exercise following a short immobilization period is detrimental to tendon properties and joint mechanics in a rat rotator cuff injury model. J Orthop Res 2010;28:841–5.
71. Soslowsky LJ, An CH, Johnston SP, et al. Geometric and mechanical properties of the coracoacromial ligament and their relationship to rotator cuff disease. Clin Orthop Relat Res 1994;(304):10–7.
72. Ward SR, Sarver JJ, Eng CM, et al. Plasticity of muscle architecture after supraspinatus tears. J Orthop Sports Phys Ther 2010;40(11):729–35.
73. Zhang S, Li H, Tao H, et al. Delayed early passive motion is harmless to shoulder rotator cuff healing in a rabbit model. Am J Sports Med 2013;41(8): 1885–92.
74. Sarver JJ, Dishowitz MI, Kim SY, et al. Transient decreases in forelimb gait and ground reaction forces following rotator cuff injury and repair in a rat model. J Biomech 2010;43(4):778–82.
75. Arndt J, Clavert P, Mielcarek P, et al. Immediate passive motion versus immobilization after endoscopic supraspinatus tendon repair: a prospective randomized study. Orthop Traumatol Surg Res 2012;98(6 Suppl):S131–8.
76. Duzgun I, Baltaci G, Atay OA. Comparison of slow and accelerated rehabilitation protocol after arthroscopic rotator cuff repair: pain and functional activity. Acta Orthop Traumatol Turc 2011;45(1):23–33.
77. Keener JD, Galatz LM, Stobbs-Cucchi G, et al. Rehabilitation following arthroscopic rotator cuff repair: a prospective randomized trial of immobilization compared with early motion. J Bone Joint Surg Am 2014;96(1):11–9.
78. Kim YS, Chung SW, Kim JY, et al. Is early passive motion exercise necessary after arthroscopic rotator cuff repair? Am J Sports Med 2012;40(4):815–21.
79. Klintberg IH, Gunnarsson AC, Svantesson U, et al. Early loading in physiotherapy treatment after full-thickness rotator cuff repair: a prospective randomized pilot-study with a two-year follow-up. Clin Rehabil 2009;23(7):622–38.
80. Lee BG, Cho NS, Rhee YG. Effect of two rehabilitation protocols on range of motion and healing rates after arthroscopic rotator cuff repair: aggressive versus limited early passive exercises. Arthroscopy 2012;28(1):34–42.
81. Parsons BO, Gruson KI, Chen DD, et al. Does slower rehabilitation after arthroscopic rotator cuff repair lead to long-term stiffness? J Shoulder Elbow Surg 2010;19(7):1034–9.
82. Yoo JH, Cho NS, Rhee YG. Effect of postoperative repair integrity on health-related quality of life after rotator cuff repair: healed versus retear group. Am J Sports Med 2013;41:2637–44.
83. Conti M, Garofalo R, Delle Rose G, et al. Post-operative rehabilitation after surgical repair of the rotator cuff. Musculoskelet Surg 2009;93(Suppl 1):S55–63.
84. Koh KH, Lim TK, Shon MS, et al. Effect of immobilization without passive exercise after rotator cuff repair: randomized clinical trial comparing four and eight weeks of immobilization. J Bone Joint Surg Am 2014;96(6):e44.
85. Chillemi C, Petrozza V, Garro L, et al. Rotator cuff re-tear or non-healing: histopathological aspects and predictive factors. Knee Surg Sports Traumatol Arthrosc 2011;19(9):1588–96.
86. Gulotta LV, Nho SJ, Dodson CC, et al. Prospective evaluation of arthroscopic rotator cuff repairs at 5 years: part I–functional outcomes and radiographic healing rates. J Shoulder Elbow Surg 2011;20(6):934–40.
87. Nho SJ, Brown BS, Lyman S, et al. Prospective analysis of arthroscopic rotator cuff repair: prognostic factors affecting clinical and ultrasound outcome. J Shoulder Elbow Surg 2009;18(1):13–20.

88. Oh JH, Kim SH, Ji HM, et al. Prognostic factors affecting anatomic outcome of rotator cuff repair and correlation with functional outcome. Arthroscopy 2009;25(1):30–9.
89. Oh JH, Kim SH, Shin SH, et al. Outcome of rotator cuff repair in large-to-massive tear with pseudoparalysis: a comparative study with propensity score matching. Am J Sports Med 2011;39(7):1413–20.
90. Brislin KJ, Field LD, Savoie FH 3rd, et al. Complications after arthroscopic rotator cuff repair. Arthroscopy 2007;23(2):124–8.
91. Huberty DP, Schoolfield JD, Brady PC, et al. Incidence and treatment of postoperative stiffness following arthroscopic rotator cuff repair. Arthroscopy 2009;25(8): 880–90.
92. Weber SC, Abrams JS, Nottage WM, et al. Complications associated with arthroscopic shoulder surgery. Arthroscopy 2002;18(2 Suppl 1):88–95.
93. Gaunt BW, McCluskey GM, Uhl TL. An electromyographic evaluation of subdividing active-assistive shoulder elevation exercises. Sports Health 2010;2(5):424–32.
94. Uhl TL, Muir TA, Lawson L. Electromyographical assessment of passive, active assistive, and active shoulder rehabilitation exercises. PM R 2010;2(2):132–41.
95. Holtby R, Razmjou H. Measurement properties of the Western Ontario rotator cuff outcome measure: a preliminary report. J Shoulder Elbow Surg 2005;14(5):506–10.
96. Kocher MS, Horan MP, Briggs KK, et al. Reliability, validity, and responsiveness of the American shoulder and elbow surgeons subjective shoulder scale in patients with shoulder instability, rotator cuff disease, and glenohumeral arthritis. J Bone Joint Surg Am 2005;87(9):2006–11.
97. Leggin BG, Michener LA, Shaffer MA, et al. The penn shoulder score: reliability and validity. J Orthop Sports Phys Ther 2006;36:138–51.
98. Michener LA, McClure PW, Sennett BJ. American shoulder and elbow surgeons standardized shoulder assessment form, patient self-report section: reliability, validity, and responsiveness. J Shoulder Elbow Surg 2002;11:587–94.
99. Wessel J, Razmjou H, Mewa Y, et al. The factor validity of the Western ontario rotator cuff index. BMC Musculoskelet Disord 2005;6:22.

Rehabilitation of the Throwing Athlete
Where We Are in 2014

Kevin E. Wilk, PT, DPT[a,b,c,*],
Todd R. Hooks, PT, ATC, OCS, SCS, NREMT-1, CSCS, CMTPT[a]

KEYWORDS

• Overhead athlete • Rehabilitation • Shoulder

KEY POINTS

• The rehabilitation program is divided into 4 phases and the progression of an athlete depends on the successful completion of each phase.
• The systematic implementation of incorporating applied stresses and forces via functional and sport-specific drills effectively allows a return to activity.
• An effective evaluation aids in the development of an optimal rehabilitation program to address the causative factors of an athlete's pathology.
• The postoperative range-of-motion (ROM) progression is based on an assessment of an athlete's quality of end feel, with an accelerated restoration warranted with a firm end feel and a slower restoration with a soft end feel.

The shoulder joint is a common site of pathology in overhead athletes. Injuries to the shoulder joint region frequently occur in the overhead thrower. Conte and colleagues[1] reported that shoulder injuries represented 27.8% of all disabled days (DLs) in professional baseball players. Based on DLs, Posner and coworkers[2] noted that pitchers experienced a 34% higher incidence injury rate compared with fielders in Major League Baseball, and when pitchers were placed on DLs for injuries to the upper extremity they remained so for a longer length of time (74.25 days vs 54.15 days). According to the National Collegiate Athletic Association Injury Surveillance System, for all injuries that required 10 plus days' time loss from 1998 to 2004, shoulder strains/tendinitis injuries equated to 8.2% of all injuries occurring during games and 16.7% of injuries during practice.[3] The shoulder has also been reported the most

[a] Champion Sports Medicine, A Physiotherapy Associates Clinic, Birmingham, AL, USA; [b] Tampa Bay Rays Baseball Team, Tampa Bay, FL, USA; [c] American Sports Medicine Institute, Birmingham, AL, USA
* Corresponding author. 805 St Vincent's Drive, G-100, Birmingham, AL 35205.
E-mail address: Kwilkpt@hotmail.com

Clin Sports Med 34 (2015) 247–261
http://dx.doi.org/10.1016/j.csm.2014.12.010
0278-5919/15/$ – see front matter © 2015 Elsevier Inc. All rights reserved.
sportsmed.theclinics.com

common injury region in high school baseball players, representing 34.2% of all injuries in pitchers and 24.9% in catchers with an overall prevalence of 17.6% for all positions.[4]

Shoulder injuries are common due to the repetitive nature of overhead throwing. There are tremendous forces placed on the glenohumeral joint as angular velocities reach 7250°/s and anterior shear forces approach 50% body weight during the throwing motion.[5–7] Athletes also generate high levels of muscular activity during the throwing motion, with forces reaching 120% maximal volitional isometric contraction.[8] Although an inherent degree of mobility is needed during the throwing motion, athletes depend on dynamic stability during the throwing motion to minimize the potential for injury. Therefore, an essential balance is needed between the extreme mobility generated during the throwing motion and the required stability to maintain joint integrity that can present as a significant challenge.

The rehabilitation program described in this article for the treatment of overhead athletes is a multiphased approach focused on a return to prior level of function via a systematic process. This program is divided into 4 phases that are designed to allow a gradual progression of exercises and implied stresses that methodically increase and build on the previous exercises to focus on restoring strength, increasing dynamic stability, and developing neuromuscular control for overhead athletes. The keys to an effective and successful restoration of function are identification of each athlete's pathologic causative factor and providing a specific treatment program to address this condition. This article describes the nonoperative rehabilitation for overhead athletes and outlines the postoperative treatment after both a superior labrum from anterior to posterior (SLAP) repair and a capsular plication procedure.

NONOPERATIVE REHABILITATION

The nonoperative rehabilitation program is designed based on the examination findings from each athlete's presentation. The program, outlined in this article, is criteria based; therefore, it is adaptable and applicable to both traumatic and nontraumatic injuries by allowing a clinician to progress each athlete throughout the rehabilitation program based on both clinical assessment and successful completion of each phase of treatment. The program is tailored to address the causative factors for each athlete based on clinical findings and is divided into 4 phases.

PHASE 1—ACUTE PHASE

The goals in this initial phase, phase 1, of the rehabilitation program are to diminish pain and inflammation, normalize motion, correct postural adaptations, normalize muscle balance, and re-establish baseline dynamic joint stability. During the acute phase of treatment, an athlete may be prescribed nonsteroidal anti-inflammatory drugs and/or local injection; however; clinically, local therapeutic modalities are used to diminish pain and inflammation, such as ice, iontophoresis, phonophoresis, and electrical stimulation. Athletes are educated on activity modification/avoidance (such as throwing, strenuous activities, and exercises) as well as sitting and standing postural education to increase subacromial space.[9]

After the abating of the acute inflammation, a rehabilitation specialist may implement the use of moist heat, warm whirlpool, and/or ultrasound aimed to increase local circulation/soft tissue extensibility to improve extensibility of the joint capsule and musculotendinous tissues along with ROM and joint mobilization techniques. Decreased electromyography (EMG) activity of 23% with a corresponding reduction of 32% external rotation (ER) force production has been documented in a painful shoulder,[10] lending credence to the importance of pain reduction to allow for restoration of normal rotator cuff recruitment.

A clinician may use soft tissue mobilization techniques with the goal of improving tissue extensibility, reduction of pain and guarding, and preparing an athlete for activities. Additionally, to diminish pain and muscle guarding via stimulation of the type 1 and 2 mechanoreceptors, active-assisted ROM (AAROM), light manual stretches, and grade 1 and 2 joint mobilizations are performed.[11–13]

During the acute phase of rehabilitation, the clinician should ensure the normalization of motion by incorporating AAROM, passive ROM, manual stretches, and mobilization techniques. Although all aspects of shoulder mobility should be assessed, it is common for overhead athletes to display a loss of internal rotation (IR) and horizontal adduction. The loss of IR is commonly described as glenohumeral IR deficit (GIRD). The loss of IR of 18° on the throwing shoulder has been implemented in shoulder and elbow injuries.[14–17] Glenohumeral IR loss has been attributed to osseous adaptations, posterior rotator cuff tightness, posterior capsule tightness, and an anteriorly tilted scapula.[1,18–23] A proper clinical assessment to differentiate between altered scapula positioning, posterior capsule tightness, and/or posterior shoulder tightness that is contributing to the diminished ROM is essential for clinicians to direct the appropriate treatment program.

A postural assessment and mobility of the scapula should be assessed because an anteriorly tilted scapula is frequently seen in overhead athletes. Postural assessment of the scapula often reveals a protracted, depressed, and anterior tilt compared with the contralateral side. This positioning can create muscle weakness and/or inhibition of the scapular retractors as a result of altered length tension relationship. In addition, pectoralis minor tightness, coracoid pain, and lower trapezius muscle weakness are often noted. The decreased flexibility of the pectoralis minor can cause neurovascular symptoms, including arm fatigue, pain, tenderness, and cyanosis, due to occlusion as the neurovascular structures pass underneath this muscle.[24,25] Lower trapezius weakness is critical in controlling scapular elevation and protraction as the arm decelerates, and weakness can result in improper mechanics and potential shoulder symptoms.[7] The pectoralis minor muscle can be assessed for tightness by having the patient stand against a wall and measuring the distance from the wall to the anterior acromial tip, with a side-to-side asymmetry greater than 3 cm considered abnormal.[26] The authors commonly perform pectoralis minor muscle stretches with the scapula placed in a retracted and posteriorly tilted position with 30° of shoulder flexion as the humerus is placed in an abducted and ER position.[27,28]

The posterior shoulder is subject to repetitive eccentrics during throwing, which can result in increased internal stiffness and decreased ROM.[29] The modified sleeper stretch (**Fig. 1**), modified cross-body horizontal adduction (**Fig. 2**), and horizontal adduction stretch with concomitant IR (**Fig. 3**) are performed to improve flexibility of the posterior shoulder.[30] The posterior capsule has been shown to exhibit significant laxity in throwers who exhibit GIRD; therefore, a proper evaluation should be performed to determine capsular mobility.[31] Mobilizations for the posterior capsule are performed parallel to the glenoid fossa in a posterior-lateral direction to increase pliability of the posterior capsule (**Fig. 4**).

During this early phase of rehabilitation, strengthening exercises are initiated with the intention of restoring muscle balance/ratios and impeding muscle atrophy.[32,33] A clinician may opt to initiate isometrics during this acute phase in the presence of excessive pain and/or soreness and progress to isotonics as tolerated. The aim of exercises is to re-establish dynamic stability; therefore, initial focus is on the innately weak posterior rotator cuff and supraspinatus.[32,33] Rhythmic stabilization (RS)

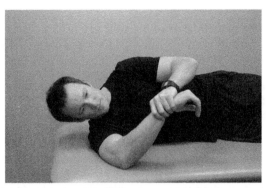

Fig. 1. Modified sleeper stretch. The athlete is rotated slightly posterior to position the shoulder in the scapular plane as IR is passively performed.

exercises are performed that initially begin for the internal rotators and external rotators with the arm in the neutral rotation as the shoulder is at 30° of abduction. Manual cueing is used to facilitate co-contraction of the internal and external rotators to provide isometric stabilization of the glenohumeral stabilization. These drills can also be initiated as the shoulder is placed in a balanced position, approximately 100° of elevation and 10° of horizontal abduction, which is beneficial because the rotator cuff and deltoid musculature resultant force vectors provide a centralized compression of the humeral head.[34,35] An athlete's arm can be placed at various angles of both ER and external elevation while applying manual cueing at various planes to facilitate recruitment of the surrounding musculature.

Proprioceptive sense can be diminished due to micro- or macrotrauma; thus, rehabilitation specialists should initiate techniques to heighten the sensory awareness of the afferent mechanoreceptors during this phase of rehabilitation.[36,37] Proprioception and enhanced functional throwing performance test scores have been shown to improve after 5-weeks' neuromuscular and proprioceptive neuromuscular facilitation (PNF) training drills that challenge the glenohumeral musculature.[38,39] RS drills are introduced for the internal and external rotators and PNF movement patterns are performed while incorporating RS to augment proprioception and dynamic stability.[32,33,35,37,40,41] Joint congruency is enhanced by facilitation of agonist and

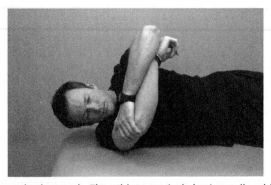

Fig. 2. Modified cross-body stretch. The athlete passively horizontally adducts the shoulder as the scapula is stabilized against the table while ER is restricted with counter pressure of the opposite forearm.

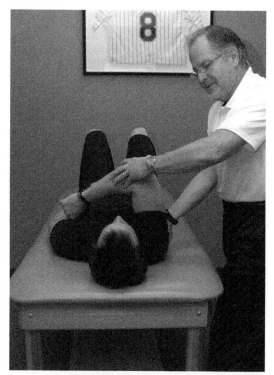

Fig. 3. Horizontal adduction with concomitant IR. The clinician performs passive horizontal abduction with concomitant IR while stabilizing the scapula as the athlete applies an IR stretch.

antagonist muscles in restoring a balance in the force couples of the shoulder joint complex.[42] Joint reproduction drills and upper extremity axial loading exercises, such as weight shifts, weight shifts on a ball, wall push-ups, and quadruped drills, are performed to stimulate the articular mechanoreceptors and aid in training proprioception during the early stage of treatment.[33,43,44]

Effective transfer of kinetic energy from the lower to the upper extremity is vital during throwing, requiring adequate mobility, stability, and strength. Core exercises are used in this phase for postural re-education, stability, and mobility of the trunk.

PHASE 2—INTERMEDIATE PHASE

The goals of phase 2 are to progress the strengthening program; increase the flexibility, mobility, and ROM of the shoulder joint complex; and enhance an athlete's neuromuscular control. An athlete can progress to the next phase once certain criteria are met; phase 2 can begin once the pain and inflammation are diminished and adequate neuromuscular control and satisfactory static stability are noted. The Thrower's Ten program designed by Wilk and colleagues[43] is based on EMG data and is implemented during this stage, allowing the progression to more aggressive isotonic strengthening activities to emphasize restoration of muscle balance.[45–53] Because the external rotators are commonly weak, side-lying shoulder ER and prone rowing into shoulder ER are prescribed due to the high EMG activity of the posterior cuff of these movements.[45]

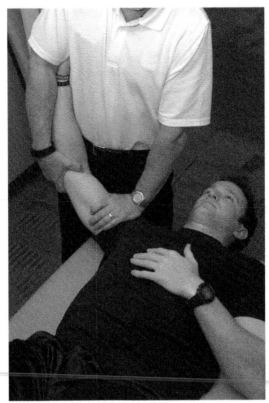

Fig. 4. Mobilizations are performed for the posterior capsule in a posterior-lateral direction.

Neuromuscular control drills are progressed as a clinician incorporates stabilization drills at the end ROM to the prior phase 1 movement drills, including PNF exercises that are performed in a full arc of a patient's available ROM. These drills serve to promote endurance training and dynamic stabilization of the rotator cuff. Manual resistance training can also be performed during this stage, allowing clinicians the ability to vary the resistance throughout the movement, incorporate concentric and eccentric movements, add RS during the exercise, and perform manual cueing for the scapular musculature.

The scapula is vital for optimal arm function because it provides proximal stability to allow for efficient distal arm mobility, and the significance of its muscular to allow for normal shoulder function has been well described by various investigators.[54–57] Wilk and Arrigo[33] formulated specific exercises designed to normalize the force couples of the scapular musculature and stimulate the proprioceptive and kinesthetic awareness to facilitate neuromuscular control of the scapulothoracic joint. The scapular retractors, protractors, and depressors are commonly emphasized due to commonly noted weakness.

Closed kinetic chain exercises are advanced to include proprioceptive drills, such as table push-ups on a ball or tilt board (**Fig. 5**), because these have been shown to generate more upper and middle trapezius and serratus anterior activity compared with performing a standard push-up exercise.[58] Stabilization drills can also be

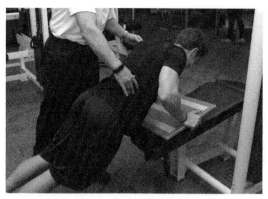

Fig. 5. Push-ups on an unstable surface with manual RSs to facilitate dynamic stability for the shoulder and core musculature.

performed when an athlete's hand is on a small ball while a clinician performs perturbation drills to the athlete's arm (**Fig. 6**).

Flexibility and ROM exercises for the shoulder joint complex are continued throughout this phase of treatment, and stretches for the trunk are incorporated into an athlete's program. Athletes can incorporate stabilization and strengthening exercises for the abdomen and lower back into the treatment program. In addition, athletes are encouraged to perform lower extremity strengthening exercises and sport-specific conditioning activities.

PHASE 3—ADVANCED STRENGTHENING PHASE

Phase 3 is designed to initiate aggressive strengthening exercises, augment power and endurance, progress functional drills, and gradually initiate throwing activities. The criteria for initiating phase 3 include full ROM, good (at least 4/5 manual muscle test) strength, minimal pain, and symmetric capsular mobility. Full shoulder ROM and flexibility should be maintained throughout this phase. Muscle fatigue has been shown to decrease neuromuscular control and diminish proprioceptive sense.[59] Therefore, athletes are further progressed with strengthening activities using the

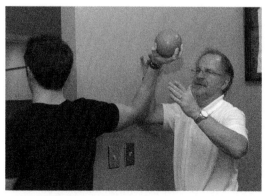

Fig. 6. Stabilization exercises as the athlete performs ball dribbles with the shoulder maintained at 90° abduction as manual stabilizations are performed.

Advanced Thrower's Ten program that incorporates high-level endurance, alternating movement patterns to further challenge shoulder girdle neuromuscular control and facilitate the rotator cuff musculature via alternating dynamic movements with sustained hold drills. The incorporation of sustained holds challenges athletes to maintain a set position while the opposite extremity performs isotonic exercises. Three sets are incorporated into each exercise, each following a sequential progression integrating bilateral isotonic movement, unilateral isotonic movement with contralateral sustained hold, and alternating isotonic/sustained hold sequencing. Athletes can be instructed to perform these exercises on a stability ball to further challenge the core (**Fig. 7**) as well as manual resistance drills to increase muscle excitation and promote endurance. Manual resistance provided by a clinician is used in seated stability ball exercises to augment muscle excitation and improve endurance of the shoulder and core musculature.

Dynamic stabilization drills, such as RS performed in a functional position, and ball throws are performed to improve proprioception and neuromuscular control. Athletes can perform stabilization techniques that include perturbations and end-range stability, including RS, by throwing a ball against a wall (**Fig. 8**), push-ups onto an unstable surface with perturbations, and ER tubing with concomitant manual resistance. In addition, these exercises can be performed on a physioball to improve dynamic stabilization of the shoulder and trunk musculature. Advanced Thrower's Ten exercises, including prone horizontal abduction and row into ER with sustained holds and alternating arm/sustained hold sequencing, are initiated to challenge the endurance of the posterior rotator cuff, scapular musculature, lumbar extensors, and gluteals. Side-lying ER, prone row, and prone horizontal manual resistance of the shoulder joint complex are used to promote increased muscular activity, neuromuscular control, and endurance, which are essential in the force production for overhead athletes.

Plyometrics are initiated to further enhance dynamic stability and proprioception as well as introduce and gradually increase functional stresses to the shoulder joint. Swanik and colleagues[60] demonstrated an enhanced joint position sense and kinesthesia as well a decreased time for peak torque generation as demonstrated with isokinetic testing. Fortun and colleagues[61] compared 8 weeks of plyometrics to conventional isotonic training and reported an increase of shoulder IR power and throwing distance. Plyometric exercises begin with a rapid prestretch eccentric contraction that stimulates the muscle spindle; followed by the amortization phase, which is the time

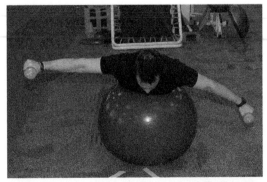

Fig. 7. Advanced Thrower's Ten exercise perform on a stability ball to facilitate stabilization of the core musculature as rotator cuff and scapular musculature endurance exercises are performed.

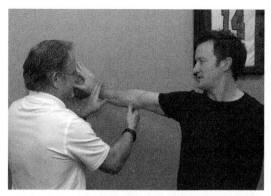

Fig. 8. Dynamic stability training with the hand placed onto a ball with the arm in the scapular plane to provide compressive forces into the glenohumeral joint as the clinician provides RSs.

between the eccentric and concentric phase. To allow an effective transfer of energy and prevent the beneficial neurologic effects of the prestretch from being dissipated as heat, this phase should be as short as possible. Athletes are instructed to coordinate the trunk and lower extremity to efficiently allow the transfer of energy into the upper extremity during the plyometric drills. Wilk and colleagues[62,63] have described a plyometric program that systematically introduces stresses on the healing tissues beginning with 2-handed drills, such as chest pass, side-to-side throws, side throws, and overhead soccer throws. On successful completion of these 2-handed drills, athletes can progress to 1-handed drills, such as standing 1-handed throws, wall dribbles, and plyometric step and throws.

Muscle fatigue has been shown to diminish proprioceptive sense and alter biomechanics; therefore, muscle endurance training should be included in the rehabilitation program for overhead athletes.[64] Kinematic and kinetic motion analysis performed by Murray and colleagues[65] reported shoulder ER and ball velocity decreased along with lead knee flexion and shoulder adduction torque once a thrower became fatigued. Muscle fatigue has been shown to attribute to superior humeral head migration on initiation of arm elevation.[66] Lyman and colleagues[67] noted the greatest predisposing factor to shoulder injury was muscle fatigue in Little League pitchers. Endurance training is performed by athletes, including wall dribbles with a Plyoball (Functional Integrated Technologies, Watsonville, California), wall arm circles, upper body cycle, and Advanced Throwers Ten exercises.

An interval throwing program (ITP) can be introduced during the third phase. The ITP was developed to gradually introduce quantity, distance, intensity, and types of throws needed to facilitate the restoration of normal throwing motions. The ITP is divided into 2 phases: phase 1 is a long toss program and phase 2 is a mound throwing program used for pitchers. Phase 1 is initiated at 45 feet (15 m) and is progressed with increased distances as well as volume of throws. Athletes are instructed to use a crow-hop method for throwing to incorporate the trunk and lower extremities while throwing with a slight arc for each prescribed distances. Fleisig and colleagues[68] reported that when pitchers were asked to throw at 50% effort, radar analysis showed it was approximately 83% of their maximum speed, and at 75% effort, the pitchers threw at 90% of their maximum effort. This study demonstrates the inherent difficulty in self-imposing velocity limitations; therefore, the authors implement a slight arc (vs throwing on a line) in the long toss program as a means to regulate the intensity of each throw and ensure that athletes are not throwing harder than needed for each distance. The long toss program is designed to gradually introduce loads and strains and should be successfully completed prior to allowing throwing from the mound. Position players can in addition begin a progressive hitting program that begins with swinging a light bat, progressing to hitting off a tee, soft toss hitting, and batting practice.

PHASE 4—RETURN TO THROWING PHASE

Phase 4 of the rehabilitation program encompasses the progression and continuation of the ITP and is designed to systemically progress athletes with throwing activates. Athletes can progress to phase 4 once full functional ROM, adequate static and dynamic stability, satisfactory muscular strength and endurance, and a satisfactory clinical examination are achieved. It is important for a clinician to continuously monitor and assess an athlete's mechanics and intensity throughout this throwing program. Position players progressed throughout the throwing program to 180 feet (60 m), whereas pitchers are progressed to 120 feet (40 m) and on successful completion can begin throwing from a wind-up on level ground at 60 feet (20 m). Pitchers can begin phase 2 of the ITP on successful completion of phase 1 of the ITP.[69] Position players during this phase are progressed with position-specific fielding drills and functional drills.

Athletes are instructed to continue with all previously described exercises and drills to maintain and improve upper extremity, core, and lower extremity strength, power, and endurance during this phase of treatment.[70–72] Additionally, athletes should be educated on a year-round conditioning program, including periodization of strength training activities and throwing to aid in the prevention of overtraining, proper conditioning prior to initiating throwing, and preparing for the upcoming season.[73] Wooden and colleagues[74] showed that a dynamic variable resistance exercise program significantly increased throwing velocity. Likewise, the throwing velocity in high school baseball players was increased using a program that incorporates a variety of resistance exercises, including plyometric training and a Thrower's Ten training.[75,76]

Rehabilitation After Arthroscopic Glenoid Labrum Procedures

The specific rehabilitation program after surgical intervention involving the glenoid labrum depends on the severity of the pathology. After a simple arthroscopic débridement of the frayed labrum, the rehabilitation program is somewhat aggressive in restoring motion and function. Full ROM is expected by 10 to 14 days postoperatively. IR and ER tubing exercises are initiated at day 10, with gradual isotonic strengthening occurring between weeks 2 and 8 with a gradual progression allowing athletes to begin an ITP at week 8 to 12.

Rehabilitation after a type II SLAP lesion is more cautious, with athletes sleeping in an immobilizer and wearing a sling in the daytime for the first 4 weeks, and, in addition, no isolated biceps strengthening is permitted for 6 to 8 weeks to allow adequate healing. ROM activity is restricted for the first 4 weeks below 90° of elevation. During the first 2 weeks, IR and ER are performed passively in the scapula plane to approximately 10° to 15° of ER and 45° of IR and are progressed to 90° of abduction at week 5 to 6. No excessive ER, extension, or abduction is allowed until week 5 to 6, when a light isotonic strengthening program is initiated. Motion is gradually increased to restore full range by 8 to 10 weeks and progressed to thrower's motion through weeks 10 to 12. Plyometric exercises are initiated at week 12 and the ITP at week 16. Return to play after surgical repair of a type II SLAP lesion occurs at approximately 9 to 11 months.

Rehabilitation After Arthroscopic Capsular Plication

Because of the inherent congenial laxity present, an overall conservative approach in restoring glenohumeral ROM is taken during the early stages of rehabilitation after capsular plication by limited ROM exercises delayed until 2 weeks after surgery. Athletes are instructed to sleep in an immobilizer and avoid elevation and ER ROM for 6 weeks and limit overhead activities for 12 weeks. ROM is limited to 90° flexion and ER performed in the scapular plane to 0° at 2 weeks, with a gradual progression to allow 145° of flexion and 45° of ER at 4 weeks. ER ROM is performed at 90° of abduction to 70° at 6 weeks as flexion is permitted to 160°. Overhead athletes continue a gradual progression of motion allowing for thrower's motion at 10 to 12 weeks.

Isometric rotator cuff and scapular exercises are integrated into the early stages of rehabilitation and progressed to light isotonics and closed-chain RS exercises to emphasize co-contraction at 4 weeks after surgery. Athletes can continue to progress the strengthening program to include the Thrower's Ten program at week 7 to 8, which is progressed to overhead dynamic strengthening at week 12. Interval sporting activities are initiated at week 16 to allow athletes to return 7 to 9 months after surgery.

SUMMARY

The overhead athlete displays unique ROM, postural, strength, and joint laxity characteristics that occur as a result of physical adaptation to the imposed stresses and demands of repetitive throwing. As a result, there are distant pathologies in this patient population described in this article. The success of the rehabilitation program depends on an accurate recognition of the underlying cause of the pathology. An effective rehabilitation program focuses on re-establishing full ROM, dynamic rotator cuff stability, and implementing a progressive resistance exercise program to fully restore strength and local muscle endurance of the rotator cuff and scapular musculature. This program evolves to include sport-specific drills and functional activities to allow a return to sport and activity.

REFERENCES

1. Conte S, Requa RK, Garrick JG. Disability days in major league baseball. Am J Sports Med 2001;29(4):431–6.
2. Posner M, Cameron KL, Wolf JM, et al. Epidemiology of major league baseball injuries. Am J Sports Med 2011;39(8):1676–80.
3. Dick R, Sauers EL, Agel J, et al. Descriptive epidemiology of collegiate men's baseball injuries: National Collegiate Athletic Association Injury Surveillance System, 1998–1989 through 2003–2004. J Athl Train 2007;42(2):183–93.
4. Collins CL, Comstock RD. Epidemiological features of high school baseball injuries in the United States, 2005–2007. Pediatrics 2008;121(6):1181–7.
5. Fleisig GS, Andrews JR, Dillman CJ, et al. Kinetics of baseball pitching with implications about injury mechanisms. Am J Sports Med 1995;23(2):233–9.
6. Fleisig GS, Barrentine SW, Escamilla RF, et al. Biomechanics of overhand throwing with implications for injuries. Sports Med 1996;21(6):421–37.
7. Escamilla RF, Barrentine SW, Fleisig GS, et al. Pitching biomechanics as a pitcher approaches muscular fatigue during a simulated baseball game. Am J Sports Med 2007;35(1):23–33.

8. Digiovine NM, Jobe FW, Pink M, et al. An electromyographic analysis of the upper extremity in pitching. J Shoulder Elbow Surg 1992;1(1):15–25.

9. Solem-Bertoft E, Thuomas KA, Westerberg CE. The influence of scapular retraction and protraction on the width of the subacromial space. An MRI study. Clin Orthop Relat Res 1993;(296):99–103.

10. Stackhouse SK, Eisennagel A, Eisennagel J, et al. Experimental pain inhibits infraspinatus activation during isometric external rotation. J Shoulder Elbow Surg 2013;22(4):478–84.

11. Matiland GD. Vertebral manipulation. 4th edition. Boston: Butterworth; 1977.

12. Wyke BD. The neurology of joints. Ann R Coll Surg Engl 1967;41(1):25–50.

13. Noyes FR, Mangine RE, Barber S. Early knee motion after open and arthroscopic anterior cruciate ligament reconstruction. Am J Sports Med 1987;15(2):149–60.

14. Wilk KE, Macrina LC, Fleisig GS, et al. Loss of internal rotation and the correlation to shoulder injuries in professional baseball pitchers. Am J Sports Med 2011;39: 329–35.

15. Myers JB, Laudner KG, Pasquale MR, et al. Glenohumeral range of motion deficits and posterior shoulder tightness in throwers with pathologic internal impingement. Am J Sports Med 2006;34:385–91.

16. Laudner KG, Myers JB, Pasquale MR, et al. Scapular dysfunction in throwers with pathologic internal impingement. J Orthop Sports Phys Ther 2006;36:485–94.

17. Dines JS, Frank JB, Akerman M, et al. Glenohumeral internal rotation deficits in baseball players with ulnar collateral ligament insufficiency. Am J Sports Med 2009;37:566–70.

18. Thomas SJ, Swanik KA, Swanik CB, et al. Internal rotation deficits affect scapular positioning in baseball players. Clin Orthop Relat Res 2010;468(6):1551–7.

19. Crockett HC, Gross LB, Wilk KE, et al. Osseous adaptation and range of motion at the glenohumeral joint in professional baseball pitchers. Am J Sports Med 2002;30:20–6.

20. Reagan KM, Meister K, Horodyski MB, et al. Humeral retroversion and its relationship to glenohumeral rotation in the shoulder of college baseball players. Am J Sports Med 2002;30:354–60.

21. Meister K, Day T, Horodyski M, et al. Rotation motion changes in the glenohumeral joint of the adolescent/little league baseball player. Am J Sports Med 2005; 33:693–8.

22. Thomas SJ, Swanik CB, Higginson JS, et al. A bilateral comparison of posterior capsule thickness and its correlation with glenohumeral range of motion and scapular upward rotation in collegiate baseball players. J Shoulder Elbow Surg 2011;20(5):708–16.

23. Kibler WB, Kuhn JE, Wilk K, et al. The disabled throwing shoulder: spectrum of pathology – 10-year update. Arthroscopy 2013;29(1):141–61.

24. Rohrer MJ, Cardullo PA, Pappas AM, et al. Axillary artery compression and thrombosis in throwing athletes. J Vasc Surg 1990;11(6):761–8.

25. Sotta RP. Vascular problems in the proximal upper extremity. Clin Sports Med 1990;9(2):379–88.

26. Kluemper M, Uhl TL, Hazelrigg H. Effects of stretching and strengthening shoulder muscles on forward shoulder posture in competitive swimmers. J Sport Rehabil 2006;15:58–70.

27. Borstad JD, Ludewig PM. Comparison of three stretches for the pectoralis minor muscle. J Shoulder Elbow Surg 2006;15(3):324–30.

28. Muraki T, Aoki M, Izumi T, et al. Lengthening of the pectoralis minor muscle during passive shoulder motions and stretching techniques: a cadaveric biomechanical study. Phys Ther 2009;89(4):333–41.

29. Butterfield TA. Eccentric exercise in vivo: strain-induced muscle damage and adaptation in a stable system. Exerc Sport Sci Rev 2010;38:51–60.

30. Wilk KE, Hooks TR, Macrina LC. The modified sleeper stretch and modified cross-body stretch to increase shoulder internal rotation range of motion in the overhead throwing athlete. J Orthop Sports Phys Ther 2013;33(8):455–67.

31. Borsa PA, Wilk KE, Jacobson JA, et al. Correlation of range of motion and gleno-humeral translation in professional baseball pitchers. Am J Sports Med 2005; 33(9):1392–9.

32. Wilk KE, Arrigo CA, Andrews JR. Current concepts: the stabilizing structures of the glenohumeral joint. J Orthop Sports Phys Ther 1997;25(6):364–79.

33. Wilk KE, Arrigo CA. An integrated approach to upper extremity exercises. Orthop Phys Ther N Am 1992;1:337–60.

34. Poppen NK, Walker PS. Forces at the glenohumeral joint in abduction. Clin Orthop Relat Res 1978;(135):165–70.

35. Walker PS, Poppen NK. Biomechanics of the shoulder joint during abduction in the plane of the scapula [proceedings]. Bull Hosp Joint Dis 1977;38(2):107–11.

36. Lephart SM, Pincivero DM, Giraldo JL, et al. The role of proprioception in the management and rehabilitation of athletic injuries. Am J Sports Med 1997; 25(1):130–7.

37. Lephart SM, Warner JJ, Borsa PA, et al. Proprioception of the shoulder joint in healthy, unstable, and surgically repaired shoulders. J Shoulder Elbow Surg 1994;3(6):371–80.

38. Uhl TL, Gieck JH, Perrin DH, et al. The correlation between shoulder joint position sense and neuromuscular control of the shoulder. J Athl Train 1999;34(2):S–10.

39. Padua DA, Guskiewicz KM, Myers JB. Effects of closed kinetic chain, open kinetic chain, and proprioceptive neuromuscular facilitation training on the shoulder. J Athl Train 1999;34(2):S–83.

40. Knott M, Voss DE. Proprioceptive neuromuscular facilitation: patterns and techniques. 2nd edition. New York: Hoever; 1968.

41. Sullivan PE, Markos PD, Minor MA. An integrated approach to therapeutic exercise: theory and clinical application. Reston (VA): Reston Publishing Company; 1982.

42. Henry TJ, Lephart SM, Stone D, et al. An electromyographic analysis of dynamic stabilizing exercises for the shoulder. J Athl Train 1998;33(Suppl):S74.

43. Wilk KE, Andrews JR, Arrigo C. Preventive and rehabilitative exercises for the shoulder and elbow. 6th edition. Birmingham (AL): American Sports Medicine Institute; 2001.

44. Wilk KE, Arrigo C, Andrews JR. Closed and open kinetic chain exercises for the upper extremity. J Sports Rehabil 1996;5:88–102.

45. Fleisig GS, Jameson GG, Cody KE, et al. Muscle activity during shoulder rehabilitation exercises. In: Proceedings of NACOB '98, The Third North American Congress on Biomechanics. Waterloo (Canada): 1998. p. 223–34.

46. Blackburn TA, McLeod WD, White B, et al. EMG analysis of posterior rotator cuff exercises. J Athl Train 1990;25:40–5.

47. Decker MJ, Hintermeister RA, Faber KJ, et al. Serratus anterior muscle activity during selected rehabilitation exercises. Am J Sports Med 1992;7(6):784–91.

48. Hintermeister RA, Lange GW, Schultheis JM, et al. Electromyographic activity and applied load during shoulder rehabilitation exercises using elastic resistance. Am J Sports Med 1998;26:210–20.

49. Jobe FW, Tibone JE, Jobe CM, et al. The shoulder in sports. In: Rockwood CA Jr, Matsen FA III, editors. The shoulder. Philadelphia: WB Saunders; 1990. p. 961–90.

50. Jobe FW, Moynes DR, Tibone JE, et al. An EMG analysis of the shoulder in pitching. A second report. Am J Sports Med 1984;12(3):218–20.
51. Pappas AM, Zawacki RM, McCarthy CF. Rehabilitation of the pitching shoulder. Am J Sports Med 1985;13(4):223–35.
52. Townsend H, Jobe FW, Pink M, et al. Electromyographic analysis of the glenohumeral muscles during a baseball rehabilitation program. Am J Sports Med 1991;19(3):264–72.
53. Moseley JB Jr, Jobe FW, Pink M, et al. EMG analysis of the scapular muscles during a shoulder rehabilitation program. Am J Sports Med 1992;29(2):128–34.
54. Kibler WB. The role of the scapula in athletic shoulder function. Am J Sports Med 1998;26(2):325–7.
55. Kibler WB. Role of the scapula in overhead throwing motion. Contemp Orthop 1991;22:525–32.
56. Paine RM. The role of the scapula in the shoulder. In: Andrews JR, Wilk KE, editors. The athlete's shoulder. New York: Churchill Livingstone; 1994. p. 495–512.
57. Davies GJ, Dickoff-Hoffman S. Neuromuscular testing and rehabilitation of the shoulder complex. J Orthop Sports Phys Ther 1993;18(2):449–58.
58. Tucker WS, Armstrong CW, Gribble PA, et al. Scapular muscle activity in overhead athletes with symptoms of secondary shoulder impingement during closed chain exercises. Arch Phys Med Rehabil 2010;91(4):550–6.
59. Carpenter JE, Blasier RB, Pellizzon GG. The effects of muscle fatigue on shoulder joint position sense. Am J Sports Med 1998;26(2):262–5.
60. Swanik KA, Lephart SM, Swanik CB, et al. The effects of shoulder plyometric training on proprioception and selected muscle performance characteristics. J Shoulder Elbow Surg 2002;11(6):579–86.
61. Fortun CM, Davies GJ, Kernozck TW. The effects of plyometric training on the shoulder internal rotators. Phys Ther 1998;78(51):S87.
62. Wilk KE. Restoration of functional motor patterns and functional testing in the throwing athlete. In: Lephart SM, Fu FH, editors. Prioprioception and neuromuscular control in joint stability. Champaign (IL): Human Kinetics; 2000. p. 415–38.
63. Wilk KE, Voight ML, Keirns MA, et al. Stretch-shortening drills for the upper extremities: theory and clinical application. J Orthop Sports Phys Ther 1993; 17(5):225–39.
64. Voight ML, Hardin JA, Blackburn TA, et al. The effects of muscle fatigue on and the relationship of arm dominance to shoulder proprioception. J Orthop Sports Phys Ther 1996;23(6):348–52.
65. Murray TA, Cook TD, Werner SL, et al. The effects of extended play on professional baseball pitchers. Am J Sports Med 2001;29(2):137–42.
66. Chen SK, Simonian PT, Wickiewicz TL, et al. Radiographic evaluation of glenohumeral kinematics: a muscle fatigue model. J Shoulder Elbow Surg 1999;8(1): 49–52.
67. Lyman SL, Fleisig GS, Osinski ED, et al. Incidence and determinants of arm injury in youth baseball pitchers: a pilot study. Med Sci Sports Exerc 1998;30(S5):S4.
68. Fleisig GS, Zheng N, Barrentine SW, et al. Kinematic and kinetic comparison of full and partial effort baseball effort baseball pitching. Presented at: American Society of Biomechanics: Proceedings of the 20th Annual Meeting. Atlanta (GA), October 17–19, 1996. p. 151–2.
69. Reinold MM, Wilk KE, Reed J, et al. Interval sport programs: guidelines for baseball, tennis, and golf. J Orthop Sports Phys Ther 2002;32(6):293–8.
70. Escamilla RF, Lewis C, Bell D, et al. Core muscle activation during Swiss ball and traditional abdominal exercises. J Orthop Sports Phys Ther 2010;40(5):265–76.

71. Escamilla RD, Yamashiro K, Paulos L, et al. Shoulder muscle activity and function in common shoulder rehabilitation exercises. Sports Med 2009;39(8):663–85.

72. Escamilla RF, Andrews JR. Shoulder muscle recruitment patterns and related biomechanics during upper extremity sports. Sports Med 2009;39(7):569–90.

73. Verkhoshansky YV. Programming and organization of training. Livonia (MI): Sportivny Press; 1988.

74. Wooden MJ, Greenfield B, Johanson M, et al. Effects of strength training on throwing velocity and shoulder muscle performance in teenage baseball players. J Orthop Sports Phys Ther 1992;15(5):223–8.

75. Escamilla RF, Ionno M, DeMahy MS, et al. Comparison of three baseball-specific 6-week training programs on throwing velocity in high school baseball players. J Strength Cond Res 2012;26(7):1767–81.

76. Escamilla RF, Fleisig GS, Yamashiro K, et al. Effects of a 4-week youth baseball conditioning program on throwing velocity. J Strength Cond Res 2010;24(12): 3247–54.

Rehabilitation of Acute Hamstring Strain Injuries

Marc A. Sherry, PT, DPT, LAT[a], Tyler S. Johnston, PT, DPT[a],
Bryan C. Heiderscheit, PT, PhD[b,c],*

KEYWORDS

- Muscle • Injury • Myotendinous • Physical therapy

KEY POINTS

- A previous hamstring strain injury is one of the most cited risks for future injury, with as many as one-third of athletes experiencing a reinjury within 2 weeks of returning to sport activity.
- A comprehensive patient evaluation assists in coming to an accurate diagnosis, providing a reasonable prognosis for time to return to sport, and helping define the rehabilitation options necessary for full recovery.
- Upon return to sport, athletes often exhibit a persistent strength deficit compared with the contralateral limb, highlighting the importance of comprehensive rehabilitation and adequate testing to determine readiness to return to sport for reducing risk of recurrent hamstring strains.

INTRODUCTION

Acute hamstring injuries are one of the most common injuries resulting in loss of time for athletes at all levels of competition.[1-8] Those involved in sports that require high sprinting speeds, such as track, football, and rugby, are especially prone to injury.[9,10] Previous literature has indicated that nearly 1 in 3 hamstring injuries will recur and that many of these would happen within the first 2 weeks on return to sport.[1,2] This high rate of recurrence may be due to a combination of ineffective rehabilitation and inadequate return to sport criteria.

Two specific injury mechanisms have been defined that seem to influence the injury location and rehabilitation requirement, high-speed running and excessive

[a] Sports Medicine, University of Wisconsin Hospital and Clinics, 621 Science Drive, Madison, WI 53711, USA; [b] Department of Orthopedics and Rehabilitation, University of Wisconsin-Madison, 1300 University Avenue, Madison, WI 53706, USA; [c] Department of Biomedical Engineering, University of Wisconsin-Madison, 1300 University Avenue, Madison, WI 53706, USA
* Corresponding author. Department of Orthopedics and Rehabilitation, University of Wisconsin-Madison, 1300 University Avenue, Madison, WI 53706.
E-mail address: heiderscheit@ortho.wisc.edu

Clin Sports Med 34 (2015) 263–284
http://dx.doi.org/10.1016/j.csm.2014.12.009
0278-5919/15/$ – see front matter © 2015 Elsevier Inc. All rights reserved.

stretching. During high-speed running, the terminal swing phase has been identified as the time of hamstring injury occurrence, most often involving biceps femoris long head.[11,12] During this phase of the gait cycle, the hamstring muscles are active while lengthening (eccentric contraction) to absorb energy to slow the advancing limb in preparation for foot contact.[13–15] These injuries typically involve the intramuscular tendon, or aponeurosis, and the surrounding tissues.[16] The second defined injury mechanism involves an overstretch, which more commonly injures the proximal free tendon of the semimembranosus.[17,18] These injuries are common to dancing and kicking activities, in which a combined hip flexion with knee extension movement occurs. Current evidence indicates that athletes with injuries involving the proximal free tendon take longer to recover, such that return to sport may be prolonged.[18] Despite the differences in mechanism, structures involved, and healing rates, current rehabilitation approaches do not differ greatly when treating high-speed running versus overstretch injuries. This topic is an area for future research and investigation.

The goals of rehabilitation for hamstring injuries are to return the athlete to sport, return to prior level of performance, and return to participation with minimal risk for reinjury.[19] As such, deficits experienced as a direct result of the injury (eg, pain, swelling, weakness, reduced range of motion) must be addressed throughout the rehabilitation process. In addition to treating the muscle injury, underlying mechanical imbalances may be corrected to reduce the risk of recurrent injuries. Previous research has identified risk factors for initial hamstring injury. Of these, modifiable risk factors include hamstring weakness, fatigue, reduced flexibility,[20–23] imbalances in hamstring eccentric and quadriceps concentric strength,[24–26] decreased quadriceps flexibility,[27] and strength and coordination deficits of the pelvis and trunk musculature.[2,28] It can be speculated that addressing these issues after hamstring injury would also likely decrease reinjury risk.

PATIENT EVALUATION OVERVIEW

Determining the exact source of injury is critical in determining the most appropriate treatment and expediting safe return to play. Considering the potential causes of posterior thigh pain, the differential diagnosis for acute hamstring muscle strain injury includes hamstring tendon avulsion, ischial apophyseal avulsion, adductor muscle strain injury, proximal hamstring tendinopathy, and referred posterior thigh pain.

Differential diagnosis
- Complete or partial tendon avulsion
  - Mechanism: Forceful overpressure with combined knee extension and hip flexion, such as failed water ski starts, slipping into the splits, or getting tackled with overpressure[29,30]
  - Demographics: Middle- to old-aged adults, men more than women
  - Common subjective findings: Athlete may report hearing a loud pop and experience significant pain and immediate loss of function
  - Common objective findings: Extensive ecchymosis, palpable defect (after hematoma has resolved), positive result of bowstring test, inability or significant difficulty performing a prone leg curl, positive findings on magnetic resonance imaging (MRI) for tendon avulsion with or without retraction[31–33]
- Hamstring muscle/aponeurosis injury
  - Mechanism: Eccentric contraction injury, likely during terminal swing phase of high-speed running

- Demographics: Athletes involved in sprint and agility sports
- Common subjective findings: Possible audible pop; complaint of sudden onset of sharp, stabbing, or twingelike pain that is well defined; usually unable to continue inciting activity[34]
- Common objective findings: Difficulty walking or running, possible bruising, pain and substantial decrease in strength with resistive testing (more severe injuries are weak in shortened and lengthened ranges, whereas less severe ones are weak only in lengthened ranges), pain and limitation in movement with active and passive knee extension testing[19,35,36]
- Hamstring proximal free tendon injury
  - Mechanism: Lengthening overstretch injury involving excessive hip flexion combined with knee extension
  - Demographics: Athletes involved in kicking sports and dance
  - Common subjective findings: Possible audible pop, complaint of sudden onset of sharp, stabbing, or twingelike pain that is very proximal[37,38]
  - Common objective findings: Difficulty walking or running, possible bruising, pain and substantial decrease in strength with resistive testing, pain and limitation in movement with active and passive knee extension testing[18]
- Ischial tuberosity/apophyseal injury
  - Mechanism: Forceful low-velocity overstretch, often with combined hip flexion and knee extension, common in dance and kicking[39,40]
  - Demographics: Young athletes with open growth plates[39]
  - Common subjective findings: Possible audible pop, deep achy pain, discomfort with sitting[39]
  - Common objective findings: Pain and weakness with strength testing, pain and potentially increased motion on active and passive knee extension testing
- High hamstring tendinopathy
  - Mechanism: No specific incident, gradual onset of pain that can vary in intensity
  - Demographics: More common in middle-aged athletes and endurance athletes[41,42]
  - Common subjective findings: Feelings of tightness or cramping, pain that is very near or at the ischial tuberosity
  - Common objective findings: Pain with minimal, if any, weakness on resistive testing; pain with minimal, if any, limitation in flexibility;[43,44] positive result in neuromobility examination, such as slump test or lower limb tension test; positive results in bent knee stretch test and Puranen-Orava test[44]
- Adductor muscle strain injury
  - Mechanism: Quick acceleration or change of direction, typically with extreme hip abduction and external rotation[45]
  - Demographics: Athletes participating in sprint or agility sports, especially those with frontal plane movements, such as soccer and hockey
  - Common subjective findings: Sudden onset of pain in the medial thigh
  - Common objective findings: Tenderness to palpation of adductor tendons because they insert on the pubic ramus, pain with resisted hip adduction, positive findings on MRI for adductor muscle/tendon injury[46]
- Referred pain to the posterior thigh
  - Mechanism: No specific incident, gradual onset of pain that can vary in intensity
  - Demographics: Generally older athletes, may have preexisting spinal conditions

- o Common subjective findings: Feelings of tightness or cramping[47,48]
- o Common objective findings: Symptoms likely to be more position, posture, or movement specific (especially prolonged postures or movements); positive result of neuromobility examination, such as slump test

Prognosis
- The mechanism of injury can provide insight into the duration of recovery
  - o Athletes with high-speed running injuries recover quicker, with return to prior level of competition in an average of 16 weeks, than those with overstretch injuries, which can take up to 50 weeks[16,18]
- Certain characteristics of the injury are important prognostic indicators and indicate longer time to recovery
  - o More proximal injury, measured as point of maximal palpation pain in centimeters distal to the ischial tuberosity, especially if it involves the free tendon[18]
  - o Larger lesion as visualized with MRI[49]
  - o Greater reduction in active range of motion on examination correlates to longer time to return to sport[35]
  - o Time to walk: More than 1 day before walking pain-free indicates greater than 3 weeks before return to sport, when compared with less than 3 weeks for those who were able to walk without pain less than 24 hours postinjury[36]

The management of acute hamstring strain injuries is described in the following sections. However, the authors thought it useful to include some general recommendations for care related to each of the sources considered during the differential diagnosis process. These recommendations are not intended to be exhaustive but rather to provide the reader with an initial direction for management.

- Complete tendon avulsion
  - o Surgical considerations for open repair of the avulsed tendon, followed by lengthy rehabilitation[33]
- Ischial tuberosity/apophyseal injury
  - o Surgical management for avulsion with more than 2 cm retraction[39]
  - o Conservative therapy similar to progressive agility and core stabilization (PATS) program if minimal or no tendon retraction is present
- Adductor muscle injury
  - o Conservative management consisting of rehabilitation and pain management[50]
- Referred pain to the posterior thigh
  - o Treatment is variable and can be composed of surgical, nonsurgical, and pharmaceutical interventions that depend on the source of pain

PHARMACOLOGIC TREATMENT OPTIONS

Nonsteroidal anti-inflammatory medications (NSAIDs) may be used during the acute phase of recovery, although evidence indicates that they are of little benefit[51] and may have a negative effect on the muscle's ability to fully recovery.[52] As a result, their use has become controversial and other analgesics, such as acetaminophen, have been suggested instead. For athletes who experience prolonged pain, a corticosteroid injection[53] may be used to reduce the acute inflammation and reduce pain. Although these options are available, many athletes are able to modulate their pain with activity modification and ice alone.

NONPHARMACOLOGIC TREATMENT OPTIONS

The primary goals of rehabilitation are to return the athlete to sport at prior level of function with a minimal risk of recurrent injury. Without adequate rehabilitation athletes may still experience altered neuromuscular control, persistent weakness, or reduced extensibility of the musculotendon unit,[4,23,54–56] which is due, in part, to residual scar tissue and adaptive changes in the biomechanics and motor patterns of sport movements after injury and return to play.[1,4,57] In addition to addressing these potential deficits, a rehabilitation program should also correct modifiable factors that may have contributed to the original injury through the application of therapeutic exercises and manual techniques, such as joint mobilizations and soft tissue mobilization.

It has been proposed that many athletes will experience a change in the force-length relationship of their hamstrings after injury. After remodeling and repair, the hamstring muscle achieves peak force at shorter lengths, which may predispose the muscle to further injury when functioning at a lengthened position.[4,58,59] Eccentric exercise can shift the peak force production to longer muscle lengths.[60] This shift in force production may help to restore optimal musculotendon length for tension production to reduce risk of injury. In addition, previously injured hamstrings display altered firing patterns,[54] with decreased peak torque production[61] and decreased eccentric strength.[23]

Although strengthening the injured hamstring muscle is commonly the focus of rehabilitation programs, a few incorporate training to address adjacent tissues.[20,22] Neuromuscular control of the lumbopelvic region has been indicated as an important component for hamstring function during sporting activities[62] and should be an integral part to a comprehensive rehabilitation program. Sherry and Best[2] demonstrated a significant decrease in hamstring injury recurrence by using PATS exercises compared with stretching and strengthening at 2 weeks and 1 year after return to sport. Indeed, athletes who performed the PATS exercises were able to return to sport sooner and had a reinjury rate less than 10%.

Neuromobilization techniques have been recommended as part of the treatment program if a positive result of slump test is found on examination.[63] For those diagnosed with grade I injury with mild disruption of muscle fibers, slump stretching has been shown to reduce time away from sport,[64] although no information is available for more severe injuries.

With the above-mentioned considerations in mind, the rehabilitation guide discussed below is proposed for treatment of grade I and II hamstring strain injuries involving the intramuscular tendon.[2,19,49] The focus for phase I is minimization of pain and edema, restoration of normal neuromuscular control at slow speed, and prevention of excessive scar formation while protecting the healing fibers from excessive lengthening. Phase II allows for increased intensity of exercise, neuromuscular training at faster speed and larger amplitudes, and the initiation of eccentric resistance training. Phase III progresses to high-speed neuromuscular training and eccentric resistance training in a lengthened position in preparation for return to sport.

PHASE I (0–4 WEEKS)
Protection
- Direct stretching of the injured hamstring should be avoided
- Crutches may be used in moderate to severe injuries
- In mild to moderate injuries, athletes should shorten their stride length to ambulate pain free

Management of pain and swelling
- Modification of activity to avoid tension on the hamstring during the acute phase
- Compression thigh wraps for moderate to severe injuries to help decrease swelling
- Slight elevation above the heart for moderate to severe injuries to help decrease swelling
- Cryotherapy
- Use of acetaminophen for pain relief as needed, avoiding NSAIDs

Therapeutic exercises
- Stationary biking for easy motion, working toward full knee extension
- Progressive agility and trunk stabilization
  - Low- to moderate-intensity side stepping
  - Low- to moderate-intensity grapevine stepping (lateral stepping with the trail leg going over the lead leg, and then under the lead leg), both directions (**Fig. 1**)
  - Low- to moderate-intensity steps forward and backward over a tape line while moving sideways
  - Single-leg stand, progressing from eyes open to eyes closed
  - Prone abdominal body bridge (performed by using abdominal and hip muscles to hold body in a face down straight plank position with the elbows and feet being the only points of contact)
  - Supine extension bridge (performed by using abdominal and hip muscles to hold the body in a supine hook lying position with the head, upper back, arms, and feet being the points of contact)
  - Side bridge (performed by using abdominal and hip muscles to hold the body in a side-lying plank position with the lower elbow and feet being the only points of contact)

Criteria for progression to the next phase
- Normal walking stride without pain
- Very-low-speed jogging without pain
- Pain-free isometric contraction against submaximal (50%–70%) resistance during prone knee flexion (90°) manual muscle test

PHASE II (2–6 WEEKS)
Protection
- Avoiding end range lengthening of hamstring while hamstring weakness is present

Management of pain and swelling
- Ice as needed for postrehabilitation soreness

Manual therapy techniques[65]
- Utilizing manual therapy to normalize indirect joint mobility or flexibility limitations
  - Normalizing ankle dorsiflexion range of motion
  - Addressing spinal mobility limitations
  - Assessing sacroiliac joint restrictions affecting pelvic mobility
  - Using soft tissue techniques (manual or self directed) to limit excessive scar tissue formation
  - Continuing to avoid direct hamstring stretches to allow fiber repair

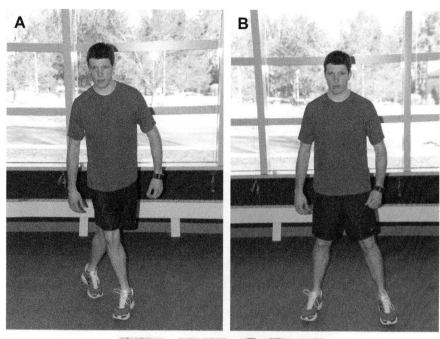

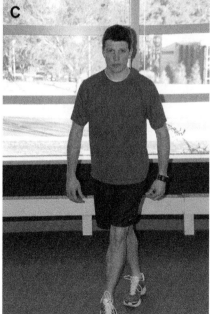

Fig. 1. Low- to moderate-intensity grapevine stepping (lateral stepping with repeated cycles of A. The trail leg going over the lead leg, B. lateral step with lead leg, and C. trail leg going under the lead leg).

Therapeutic exercises
- Progressive agility and trunk stabilization
  - Moderate- to high-intensity side stepping

- Moderate- to high-intensity grapevine stepping
- Moderate- to high-intensity steps forward and backward while moving sideways
- Single-leg stand windmill touches (performed by standing on 1 leg, then rotating the trunk and flexing the hips to bring the hand down in front of the lower leg)
- Supine bent knee bridge walk out (**Fig. 2**)

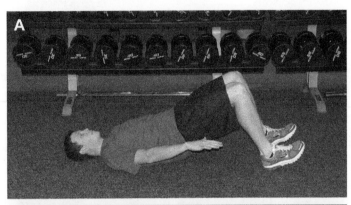

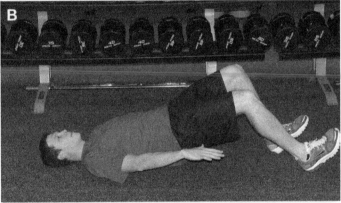

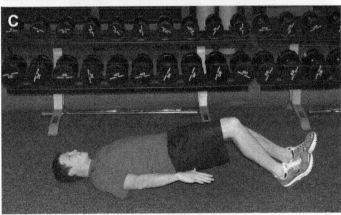

Fig. 2. Supine bent knee bridge walk out. Start in (*A*) supine bridge position and (*B* and *C*) perform a gradual movement of feet away from hips, while maintaining bridge position.

- Pushup stabilization with trunk rotation (performed by starting at the top of a full pushup, then maintaining this position with 1 hand while rotating the chest toward the side of the hand that is being lifted to point toward the ceiling, and then pausing and returning to the starting position)
- Side plank stabilization with trunk rotation (performed by starting in an extended arm side plank support with the top arm reaching up toward the ceiling, then while maintaining the hip height rotate through the trunk and neck to reach the top arm under and through, pause and then return to the start position) (**Fig. 3**)
- Fast feet in place (performed by jogging in place with increasing velocity, picking the foot only a few inches off the ground)
- High to low (**Fig. 4**) and low to high (**Fig. 5**) wood chops
- Neuromobilization[64] techniques if the patient displays adverse limb tension[63]
- Progressive balance training with balance board and unstable surface
- Eccentric resistance training
  - The Diver (**Fig. 6**) as described by Askling[66]
  - The Glider (**Fig. 7**)as described by Askling[66]

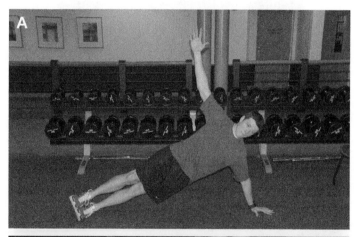

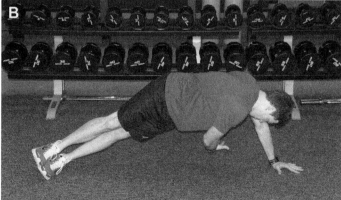

Fig. 3. Side plank stabilization with trunk rotation (performed by (*A*) starting in an extended arm side plank support with the top arm reaching up toward the ceiling, then (*B*) while maintaining the hip height rotate through the trunk and neck to reach the top arm under and through, pause and then return to the start position).

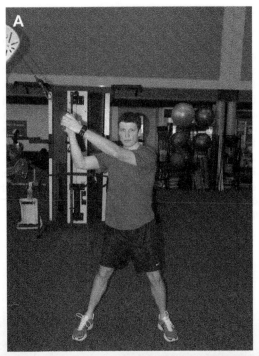

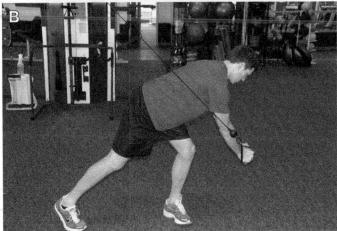

Fig. 4. High to low wood chops. Using resistance cable or elastic tubing, begin with (*A*) trunk extended and arms over one shoulder, then (*B*) rotate and flex trunk toward opposite side.

Criteria for progression to the next phase
- Full strength without pain during 1 repetition maximum isometric contraction in prone position with knee flexed to 30°
- Forward and backward jogging at 50% speed with no pain

PHASE III (4–8 WEEKS AND BEYOND)
Protection
- Avoiding full intensity if pain/tightness/stiffness is present

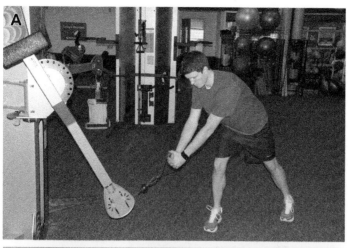

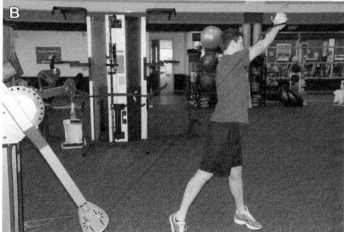

Fig. 5. Low to high wood chops. Using resistance cable or elastic tubing, begin with (*A*) trunk flexed and rotated to one side, then (*B*) rotate and extend trunk toward opposite shoulder.

Management of pain and swelling
- Use of ice as needed for postrehabilitation or practice soreness

Manual therapy techniques
- Continuing to address indirect limitations in mobility
- Manual, instrumented, or self-directed soft tissue mobilization may be more aggressively used if there is concern for excessive scar tissue formation
- No longer limited in range of motion, so stretching and flexibility for the musculotendinous unit should be initiated

Therapeutic exercises
- Progressive agility and trunk stabilization; sport-specific and agility drills should be emphasized, with a focus on quick direction changes and technique training
  - Dynamic agility drills
    - Side shuffle

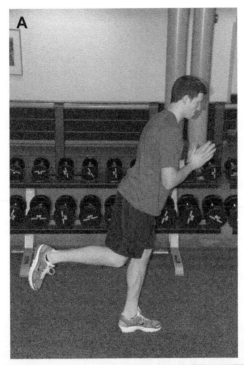

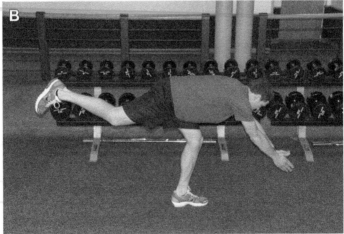

Fig. 6. The Diver. (*A*) Start by standing on the injured side, then (*B*) simultaneously flex the trunk and shoulders and extend the contralateral hip and knee, while maintaining a level pelvis.

- Carioca
- Boxer shuffles
- A skips
- B skips
- Forward and backward running
- Repetitive hop for distance

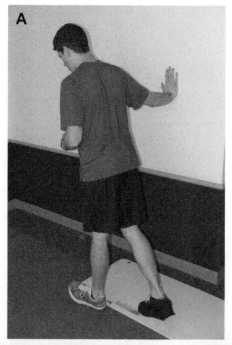

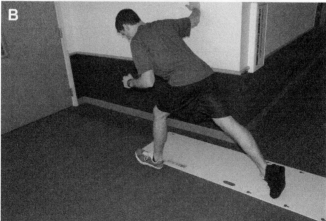

Fig. 7. The Glider. (*A*) Start with an upright trunk and majority of weight on injured leg on stable surface with one hand support, then (*B*) glide backward on opposite leg and stop before pain occurs. Return to start position using arms only.

- ○ Eccentric hamstring training at end range of motion
    - ■ Single-leg chair bridge (**Fig. 8**)
    - ■ Single-limb windmill touches with dumbbells (**Fig. 9**)
    - ■ Lunge walk with trunk rotation, opposite hand dumbbell toe touch (**Fig. 10**)
    - ■ T-lift lunge walk (**Fig. 11**)
    - ■ Single-leg dead lift
    - ■ Single-leg dumbbell hang clean

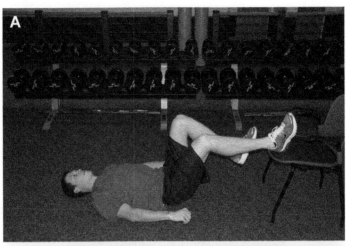

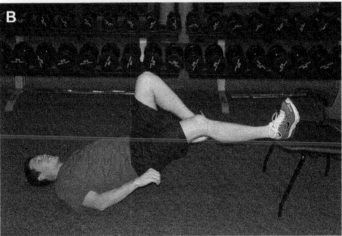

Fig. 8. Single-leg chair bridge. (*A*) Starting with 1 leg on stationary object, (*B*) raise hips and pelvis off ground.

- Modified Nordic curls using resistance cables to facilitate performance of exercise through a greater range of motion (**Fig. 12**)

Criteria for return to sport
- Pain-free palpation over the site of injury
- Full concentric and eccentric strength of the hamstrings (compared with the uninjured side) tested in a lengthened position; if using isokinetic strength testing, bilateral deficit should be less than 5%[67]
- Full concentric and eccentric muscular endurance of the hamstrings (when compared with the uninjured side), tested in a lengthened position; if using isokinetic strength testing, bilateral deficit should be less than 5%[67]
- Symmetric neuromotor properties (based on isokinetic testing)
  ○ Angle of peak torque within 5°[61]
  ○ Time to peak torque within 10% side to side[54]
- No fear or kinesiophobia, as measured by the hamstring active test, or Askling H-test[68]

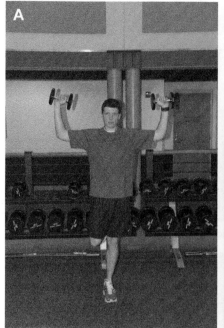 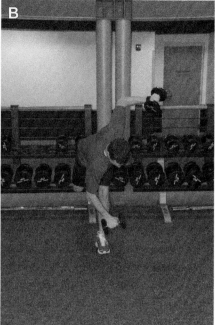

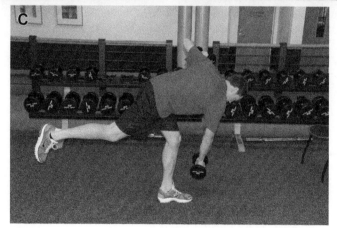

Fig. 9. Single-limb windmill touches with dumbbells. Begin in (*A*) single-limb stance position with dumbbells overhead and (*B*) perform windmill motion under control with end position of (*C*) touching dumbbell near floor.

- High-speed running drills without experiencing pain or discomfort[66]

If patients are not making consistent improvements in strength or progression toward return to play by 12 to 14 weeks, they should be reevaluated by the physician. Adjuncts to rehabilitation may be considered at this time, such as platelet-rich plasma injection, dry needling, or cortisone injection.

SURGICAL TREATMENT OPTIONS

Surgical options for the treatment of an acute hamstring strain or tear are limited at this time. The nature of the injury and the technical difficulties of surgery prevent primary

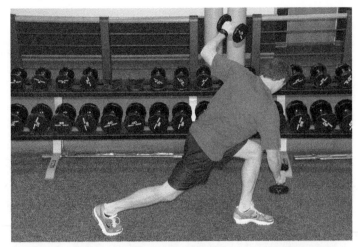

Fig. 10. Lunge walk with trunk rotation, opposite hand dumbbell toe touch.

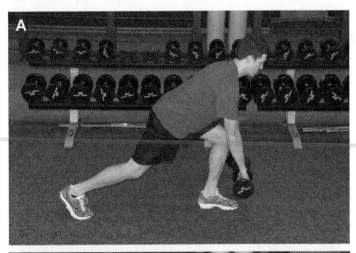

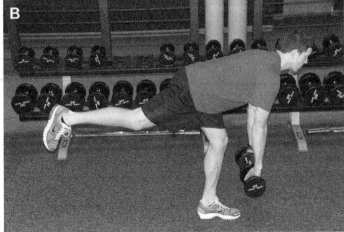

Fig. 11. T-lift lunge walk. Start in (*A*) forward lunge position, then (*B*) lift one leg off ground while maintaining a level pelvis.

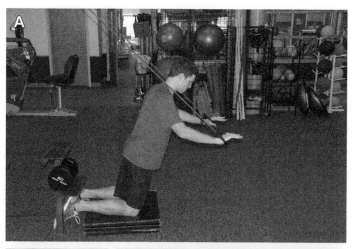

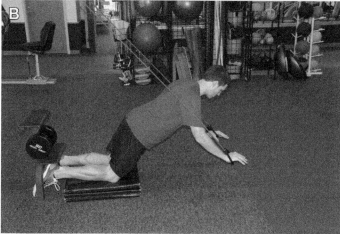

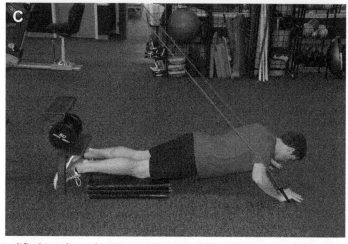

Fig. 12. Modified Nordic curls using resistance cables to facilitate performance of exercise through a greater range of motion. From (*A*) starting position, (*B*) lean trunk forward without flexing at the hips or low back until (*C*) maximum motion occurs. Return to starting position using push from floor and cables.

repair of the tissue from being a valid option. In some cases in which excessive scar tissue may be entrapping the sciatic nerve or creating intermuscular adhesions, surgical neurolysis or scar debridement may be an option.

TREATMENT RESISTANCE/COMPLICATIONS

One potential complication during the rehabilitation process is symptom exacerbation because of exercise intensity and range of motion. All exercises should be progressed based on the athlete's tolerance, and progression should be slowed if the athlete reports pain, increased stiffness, or anxiety with movement. A rehabilitation specialist's clinical decision making is paramount for safe progression of exercises without risking undue harm to the recovering athlete.

EVALUATION OF OUTCOME AND LONG-TERM RECOMMENDATIONS

Based on reinjury rates and the fact that abnormalities in MRI persist after being clinically asymptomatic, the authors recommend that athletes continue a program for performance enhancement and prevention of reinjury for the rest of the season and through the following off-season.[49] In addition, before starting their next season, the athletes should be screened for potential muscle imbalances, compensations, or weaknesses that would predispose them to other injuries.[2,61,69] Such off-season programs should include:

- Single-leg balance exercises and perturbation-type exercises
- Dynamic agility drills
- Eccentric hamstring strengthening, especially in lengthened positions
- Core and trunk stabilizing exercises

The Functional Assessment Scale for Acute Hamstring Injuries has been shown to be a reliable tool in documenting outcomes for acute hamstring injuries. The ability of this scale to determine readiness to return to play has not yet been validated.[70]

SUMMARY/DISCUSSION

Acute hamstring injuries continue to be one of the most common reasons for loss of playing time in athletes. By obtaining a complete subjective report with emphasis on injury mechanism and by performing a comprehensive physical evaluation, the rehabilitation specialist can determine the most accurate diagnosis and appropriate pathway for care. Adequate rehabilitation should address deficits in muscle strength, flexibility, neuromuscular control, and lumbopelvic stability, as these have been shown to allow the athlete to return to sport sooner and with less chance of reinjury.[2,49] Throughout the rehabilitation process, additional interventions should be used to address modifiable risk factors and should be continued through the off-season to decrease the risk for recurrent injury.

REFERENCES

1. Orchard J, Best TM. The management of muscle strain injuries: an early return versus the risk of recurrence. Clin J Sport Med 2002;12(1):3–5.
2. Sherry MA, Best TM. A comparison of 2 rehabilitation programs in the treatment of acute hamstring strains. J Orthop Sports Phys Ther 2004;34(3):116–25.
3. Sherry M. Examination and treatment of hamstring related injuries. Sports Health 2012;4(2):107–14.

4. Sanfilippo JL, Silder A, Sherry MA, et al. Hamstring strength and morphology progression after return to sport from injury. Med Sci Sports Exerc 2013;45(3): 448–54.
5. Marshall SW, Hamstra-Wright KL, Dick R, et al. Descriptive epidemiology of collegiate women's softball injuries: National Collegiate Athletic Association Injury Surveillance System, 1988–1989 through 2003–2004. J Athl Train 2007;42(2): 286–94.
6. Shankar PR, Fields SK, Collins CL, et al. Epidemiology of high school and collegiate football injuries in the United States, 2005–2006. Am J Sports Med 2007; 35(8):1295–303.
7. Price RJ, Hawkins RD, Hulse MA, et al. The Football Association Medical Research Programme: an audit of injuries in academy youth football. Br J Sports Med 2004;38(4):466–71.
8. Canale ST, Cantler ED Jr, Sisk TD, et al. A chronicle of injuries of an American intercollegiate football team. Am J Sports Med 1981;9(6):384–9.
9. Feeley BT, Kennelly S, Barnes RP, et al. Epidemiology of National Football League training camp injuries from 1998 to 2007. Am J Sports Med 2008;36(8):1597–603.
10. Orchard J, Seward H. Epidemiology of injuries in the Australian Football League, seasons 1997–2000. Br J Sports Med 2002;36(1):39–44.
11. Heiderscheit BC, Hoerth DM, Chumanov ES, et al. Identifying the time of occurrence of a hamstring strain injury during treadmill running: a case study. Clin Biomech (Bristol, Avon) 2005;20(10):1072–8.
12. Schache AG, Wrigley TV, Baker R, et al. Biomechanical response to hamstring muscle strain injury. Gait Posture 2009;29(2):332–8.
13. Chumanov ES, Heiderscheit BC, Thelen DG. The effect of speed and influence of individual muscles on hamstring mechanics during the swing phase of sprinting. J Biomech 2007;40(16):3555–62.
14. Thelen DG, Chumanov ES, Best TM, et al. Simulation of biceps femoris musculotendon mechanics during the swing phase of sprinting. Med Sci Sports Exerc 2005;37(11):1931–8.
15. Chumanov ES, Heiderscheit BC, Thelen DG. Hamstring musculotendon dynamics during stance and swing phases of high-speed running. Med Sci Sports Exerc 2011;43(3):525–32.
16. Askling CM, Tengvar M, Saartok T, et al. Acute first-time hamstring strains during high-speed running: a longitudinal study including clinical and magnetic resonance imaging findings. Am J Sports Med 2007;35(2):197–206.
17. Askling C, Saartok T, Thorstensson A. Type of acute hamstring strain affects flexibility, strength, and time to return to pre-injury level. Br J Sports Med 2006;40(1): 40–4.
18. Askling CM, Tengvar M, Saartok T, et al. Acute first-time hamstring strains during slow-speed stretching: clinical, magnetic resonance imaging, and recovery characteristics. Am J Sports Med 2007;35(10):1716–24.
19. Heiderscheit BC, Sherry MA, Silder A, et al. Hamstring strain injuries: recommendations for diagnosis, rehabilitation, and injury prevention. J Orthop Sports Phys Ther 2010;40(2):67–81.
20. Agre JC. Hamstring injuries. Proposed aetiological factors, prevention, and treatment. Sports Med 1985;2(1):21–33.
21. Clark RA. Hamstring injuries: risk assessment and injury prevention. Ann Acad Med Singapore 2008;37(4):341–6.
22. Worrell TW. Factors associated with hamstring injuries. An approach to treatment and preventative measures. Sports Med 1994;17(5):338–45.

23. Opar DA, Williams MD, Timmins RG, et al. The effect of previous hamstring strain injuries on the change in eccentric hamstring strength during preseason training in elite Australian footballers. Am J Sports Med 2014. [Epub ahead of print].

24. Arnason A, Andersen TE, Holme I, et al. Prevention of hamstring strains in elite soccer: an intervention study. Scand J Med Sci Sports 2008;18(1):40–8.

25. Croisier JL, Ganteaume S, Binet J, et al. Strength imbalances and prevention of hamstring injury in professional soccer players: a prospective study. Am J Sports Med 2008;36(8):1469–75.

26. Yeung SS, Suen AM, Yeung EW. A prospective cohort study of hamstring injuries in competitive sprinters: preseason muscle imbalance as a possible risk factor. Br J Sports Med 2009;43(8):589–94.

27. Gabbe BJ, Bennell KL, Finch CF, et al. Predictors of hamstring injury at the elite level of Australian football. Scand J Med Sci Sports 2006;16(1):7–13.

28. Cameron ML, Adams RD, Maher CG, et al. Effect of the HamSprint Drills training programme on lower limb neuromuscular control in Australian football players. J Sci Med Sport 2009;12(1):24–30.

29. Chakravarthy J, Ramisetty N, Pimpalnerkar A, et al. Surgical repair of complete proximal hamstring tendon ruptures in water skiers and bull riders: a report of four cases and review of the literature. Br J Sports Med 2005;39(8):569–72.

30. Sallay PI, Friedman RL, Coogan PG, et al. Hamstring muscle injuries among water skiers. Functional outcome and prevention. Am J Sports Med 1996;24(2): 130–6.

31. Konan S, Haddad F. Successful return to high level sports following early surgical repair of complete tears of the proximal hamstring tendons. Int Orthop 2010; 34(1):119–23.

32. Sarimo J, Lempainen L, Mattila K, et al. Complete proximal hamstring avulsions: a series of 41 patients with operative treatment. Am J Sports Med 2008;36(6): 1110–5.

33. Wood DG, Packham I, Trikha SP, et al. Avulsion of the proximal hamstring origin. J Bone Joint Surg Am 2008;90(11):2365–74.

34. Mueller-Wohlfahrt HW, Haensel L, Mithoefer K, et al. Terminology and classification of muscle injuries in sport: the Munich consensus statement. Br J Sports Med 2013;47(6):342–50.

35. Malliaropoulos N, Isinkaye T, Tsitas K, et al. Reinjury after acute posterior thigh muscle injuries in elite track and field athletes. Am J Sports Med 2011;39(2): 304–10.

36. Warren P, Gabbe BJ, Schneider-Kolsky M, et al. Clinical predictors of time to return to competition and of recurrence following hamstring strain in elite Australian footballers. Br J Sports Med 2010;44(6):415–9.

37. Askling CM, Tengvar M, Saartok T, et al. Proximal hamstring strains of stretching type in different sports: injury situations, clinical and magnetic resonance imaging characteristics, and return to sport. Am J Sports Med 2008;36(9):1799–804.

38. Cohen S, Bradley J. Acute proximal hamstring rupture. J Am Acad Orthop Surg 2007;15(6):350–5.

39. Gidwani S, Bircher MD. Avulsion injuries of the hamstring origin - a series of 12 patients and management algorithm. Ann R Coll Surg Engl 2007;89(4):394–9.

40. Wootton JR, Cross MJ, Holt KW. Avulsion of the ischial apophysis. The case for open reduction and internal fixation. J Bone Joint Surg Br 1990;72(4):625–7.

41. Cacchio A, Rompe JD, Furia JP, et al. Shockwave therapy for the treatment of chronic proximal hamstring tendinopathy in professional athletes. Am J Sports Med 2011;39(1):146–53.

42. Lempainen L, Sarimo J, Mattila K, et al. Proximal hamstring tendinopathy: results of surgical management and histopathologic findings. Am J Sports Med 2009; 37(4):727–34.
43. Lempainen L, Sarimo J, Mattila K, et al. Distal tears of the hamstring muscles: review of the literature and our results of surgical treatment. Br J Sports Med 2007; 41(2):80–3 [discussion: 83].
44. Puranen J, Orava S. The hamstring syndrome. A new diagnosis of gluteal sciatic pain. Am J Sports Med 1988;16(5):517–21.
45. Maffey L, Emery C. What are the risk factors for groin strain injury in sport? a systematic review of the literature. Sports Med 2007;37(10):881–94.
46. Nicholas SJ, Tyler TF. Adductor muscle strains in sport. Sports Med 2002;32(5): 339–44.
47. Brunker P, editor. Clinical sports medicine. 2nd edition. Sydney (Australia): The McGraw-Hill Compainies; 2001.
48. Fredericson M, Moore W, Guillet M, et al. High hamstring tendinopathy in runners: meeting the challenges of diagnosis, treatment, and rehabilitation. Phys Sportsmed 2005;33(5):32–43.
49. Silder A, Sherry MA, Sanfilippo J, et al. Clinical and morphological changes following 2 rehabilitation programs for acute hamstring strain injuries: a randomized clinical trial. J Orthop Sports Phys Ther 2013;43(5):284–99.
50. Tyler TF, Nicholas SJ, Campbell RJ, et al. The effectiveness of a preseason exercise program to prevent adductor muscle strains in professional ice hockey players. Am J Sports Med 2002;30(5):680–3.
51. Mishra DK, Fridén J, Schmitz MC, et al. Anti-inflammatory medication after muscle injury. A treatment resulting in short-term improvement but subsequent loss of muscle function. J Bone Joint Surg Am 1995;77(10):1510–9.
52. Rahusen FT, Weinhold PS, Almekinders LC. Nonsteroidal anti-inflammatory drugs and acetaminophen in the treatment of an acute muscle injury. Am J Sports Med 2004;32(8):1856–9.
53. Zissen MH, Wallace G, Stevens KJ, et al. High hamstring tendinopathy: MRI and ultrasound imaging and therapeutic efficacy of percutaneous corticosteroid injection. AJR Am J Roentgenol 2010;195(4):993–8.
54. Sole G, Milosavljevic S, Nicholson H, et al. Altered muscle activation following hamstring injuries. Br J Sports Med 2012;46(2):118–23.
55. Silder A, Thelen DG, Heiderscheit BC. Effects of prior hamstring strain injury on strength, flexibility, and running mechanics. Clin Biomech (Bristol, Avon) 2010; 25(7):681–6.
56. Silder A, Reeder SB, Thelen DG. The influence of prior hamstring injury on lengthening muscle tissue mechanics. J Biomech 2010;43(12):2254–60.
57. Silder A, Heiderscheit BC, Thelen DG, et al. MR observations of long-term musculotendon remodeling following a hamstring strain injury. Skeletal Radiol 2008; 37(12):1101–9.
58. Brockett CL, Morgan DL, Proske U. Predicting hamstring strain injury in elite athletes. Med Sci Sports Exerc 2004;36(3):379–87.
59. Proske U, Morgan DL, Brockett CL, et al. Identifying athletes at risk of hamstring strains and how to protect them. Clin Exp Pharmacol Physiol 2004;31(8):546–50.
60. Brockett CL, Morgan DL, Proske U. Human hamstring muscles adapt to eccentric exercise by changing optimum length. Med Sci Sports Exerc 2001;33(5):783–90.
61. Sole G, Milosavljevic S, Nicholson HD, et al. Selective strength loss and decreased muscle activity in hamstring injury. J Orthop Sports Phys Ther 2011; 41(5):354–63.

62. Orchard J, Best TM, Verrall GM. Return to play following muscle strains. Clin J Sport Med 2005;15(6):436–41.

63. Turl SE, George KP. Adverse neural tension: a factor in repetitive hamstring strain? J Orthop Sports Phys Ther 1998;27(1):16–21.

64. Kornberg C, Lew P. The effect of stretching neural structures on grade one hamstring injuries. J Orthop Sports Phys Ther 1989;10(12):481–7.

65. Hoskins W, Pollard H. Hamstring injury management–part 2: treatment. Man Ther 2005;10(3):180–90.

66. Askling CM, Tengvar M, Tarassova O, et al. Acute hamstring injuries in Swedish elite sprinters and jumpers: a prospective randomised controlled clinical trial comparing two rehabilitation protocols. Br J Sports Med 2014;48(7):532–9.

67. Croisier JL, Forthomme B, Namurois MH, et al. Hamstring muscle strain recurrence and strength performance disorders. Am J Sports Med 2002;30(2): 199–203.

68. Askling CM, Nilsson J, Thorstensson A. A new hamstring test to complement the common clinical examination before return to sport after injury. Knee Surg Sports Traumatol Arthrosc 2010;18(12):1798–803.

69. Askling C, Karlsson J, Thorstensson A. Hamstring injury occurrence in elite soccer players after preseason strength training with eccentric overload. Scand J Med Sci Sports 2003;13(4):244–50.

70. Malliaropoulos N, Korakakis V, Christodoulou D, et al. Development and validation of a questionnaire (FASH-Functional Assessment Scale for Acute Hamstring Injuries): to measure the severity and impact of symptoms on function and sports ability in patients with acute hamstring injuries. Br J Sports Med 2014;48(22): 1607–12.

Clinical Strategies for Addressing Muscle Weakness Following Knee Injury

Brian Pietrosimone, PhD, ATC[a],*, J. Troy Blackburn, PhD, ATC[a],
Matthew S. Harkey, MS, ATC[b], Brittney A. Luc, MS, ATC[b],
Derek N. Pamukoff, MS[b], Joe M. Hart, PhD, ATC[c]

KEYWORDS

- Disinhibitory modalities • Transcutaneous electrical nerve stimulation
- Transcranial magnetic stimulation • Electromyographic biofeedback

KEY POINTS

- Quadriceps strength may be a major contributor to disability and the progression of chronic joint disease following acute knee injury and in patients with knee osteoarthritis.
- Traditional therapeutic exercise may not target the neuromuscular origins of muscle weakness, leading to persistent strength deficits long after the initial injury and return to activity.
- Augmenting strength training with disinhibitory modalities or by using alternative strengthening techniques may help maximize strength gains from therapeutic exercise-based rehabilitation.

INTRODUCTION

Lower extremity muscle weakness is common following acute and chronic knee joint injury, and often persists long after the injury has occurred. Persistent muscle weakness following joint injury is dangerous because

1. Muscle weakness may negatively affect physical performance, disability, and willingness to engage in physical activity.
2. Muscle weakness may contribute in the progression of acute to chronic joint injury.

This article discusses the emerging evidence and novel rehabilitation strategies for maximizing strength gains following acute knee injury or surgery, and in patients with knee osteoarthritis.

---

[a] Department of Exercise and Sport Science, University of North Carolina at Chapel Hill, 209 Fetzer Hall, CB#8700, Chapel Hill, NC 27599-8700, USA; [b] Human Movement Sciences, University of North Carolina at Chapel Hill, 209 Fetzer Hall, CB#8700, Chapel Hill, NC 27599-8700, USA; [c] Department of Kinesiology, University of Virginia, 210 Emmet Street South, PO Box 4000407, Charlottesville, VA 22904, USA
* Corresponding author.
E-mail address: brian@unc.edu

Clin Sports Med 34 (2015) 285–300
http://dx.doi.org/10.1016/j.csm.2014.12.003
0278-5919/15/$ – see front matter © 2015 Elsevier Inc. All rights reserved.

EVIDENCE FOR PERSISTENT MUSCLE WEAKNESS FOLLOWING KNEE INJURY

Quadriceps muscle weakness is of great clinical concern because the quadriceps is critical for allowing people to complete activities of daily living.[1] Persistent quadriceps muscle weakness has been demonstrated in patients following anterior cruciate ligament (ACL) injury and ACL reconstructed (ACL-R) in subacute phases years after injury.[2] Quadriceps strength is critical in predicting self-reported disability in younger patients with a history or ACL injury. Quadriceps strength alone predicts 61% of the variance in self-reported function in ACL-R patients, indicating that ACL-R patients with stronger quadriceps are associated with less disability a mean of 4.5 years following surgery.[3] Interlimb deficits in quadriceps strength have been reported from less than 1 month and up to 4 years after arthroscopic meniscectomy.[4] Altered gait biomechanics are common in patients with persistent muscle weakness following acute joint injury.[5–7] ACL-injured or ACL-R patients demonstrate more extended or stiffened knee joint angles during walking gait,[6,8,9] potentially due to the inability to adequately eccentrically activate the quadriceps during the stance phase of gait.[10] A more extended knee at initial foot contact and during midstance of gait may alter proper energy attenuation, leading to a high rate of impulsive loading, which is known to damage cartilage cells.[11,12] Impulsive loading has been identified in patients with ACL injury[7] as well as patients with knee osteoarthritis,[13] suggesting that impulsive loading may be a factor in the development of osteoarthritis following acute injury.[14]

Quadriceps strength predicts disease severity, disability, and quality of life in a variety of patient populations with chronic disease such as chronic obstructive pulmonary disease (COPD),[15,16] coronary artery disease,[17] and diabetes.[18] Furthermore, quadriceps strength predicts mortality rates in patients with COPD.[19] It is not known if diminished quadriceps strength precedes decrements in quality of life in patients with chronic disease; however, it is hypothesized that inability to effectively ambulate may increase disability related to multiple diseases.[20] Quadriceps strength may play a more direct role in the disability associated with chronic joint conditions. Quadriceps strength and neuromuscular activation predict disability in patients with knee osteoarthritis.[21] Additionally, quadriceps strength predicts approximately 20% of the variance in self-reported leisure-time exercise in people with knee osteoarthritis.[22] Patients that reported engaging in less frequent or less intense leisure-time exercise may have weaker quadriceps compared with knee osteoarthritis patients that report engaging in more leisure-time exercise. Maximizing strength gains during rehabilitation is important for all stages of joint injury. Establishing symmetric bilateral strength early following knee injury or in the beginning stages of osteoarthritis may benefit long-term joint heath.

AUGMENTING TRADITIONAL STRENGTH TRAINING WITH DISINHIBITORY INTERVENTIONS

Traditional rehabilitation and strengthening exercises are often ineffective in individuals with knee conditions, likely due to underlying neural adaptations driving the development of muscular weakness.[23,24] Mikesky and colleagues[24] reported that a 12-week strength training program improved hamstring strength but did not influence quadriceps strength in individuals with knee osteoarthritis, suggesting that neuromuscular mechanisms selectively limited the efficacy of quadriceps strengthening. Hurley and colleagues[23] reported similar results in individuals with traumatic knee injuries (eg, ACLR, meniscectomy) and observed that neuromuscular deficits influenced the efficacy of strength training because those with less neuromuscular deficit demonstrated greater quadriceps strength but those with greater neuromuscular deficit did not.

These findings suggest that neuromuscular quadriceps deficits impede rehabilitation of knee conditions by limiting the efficacy of quadriceps strengthening.

Historically, arthrogenic muscle inhibition has been described as the reflexive neuromuscular inhibition of uninjured musculature surrounding an injured joint.[25] More recent experiments have demonstrated that neuromuscular inhibition is also affected by changes in function of the primary motor cortex,[26] suggesting that altered descending motor information may play a role in neuromuscular inhibition. Neuromuscular inhibition is likely an acute protective response following injury but it may persist following traditional therapeutic exercise. Long-term outcomes from traditional therapeutic exercise may be improved by incorporating novel rehabilitation methods that target neuromuscular alterations in conjunction with therapeutic exercise to elicit greater strength gains at various stages of joint injury (acute, subacute, and chronic).

Muscle contraction is generated by 2 major mechanisms: (1) voluntary control via excitation of the motor cortex of the brain or (2) reflexively through excitation of spinal reflexive pathways. Patients who recover neuromuscular activation following ACL-R demonstrate more excitable spinal reflexive pathways than ACL-R patients who exhibit persistent deficits in neuromuscular activation.[27] Additionally, ACL-R patients with persistent deficits in neuromuscular activation have less excitable neural pathways arising from the primary motor cortex of the brain, suggesting that altered excitability of regions in the brain may contribute to muscle weakness following knee injury.[27] Specifically targeting neuromuscular inhibition by upregulating spinal reflex or cortical excitability in conjunction with traditional therapeutic exercise may maximize strength gains (**Fig. 1**). Decreasing neuromuscular inhibition predicts 47% of the variance in improved strength for people with knee osteoarthritis.[28]

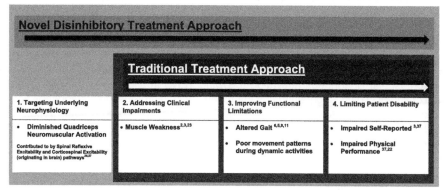

Fig. 1. A novel disinhibitory treatment approach. A continuum of clinical goals that begin with targeting underlying neurophysiological impairments (eg, arthrogenic muscle inhibition) and progress to addressing limitations in patient disability. Although steps can be addressed simultaneously, the authors propose that each subsequent step (2–4) builds on clinical improvements made in the previous steps. Traditional rehabilitation (*black box*) care is initiated by treating clinical impairments (step 2) of muscle weakness without altering the underlying neurophysiological impairments. Novel disinhibitory treatment approach (*gray box*) targets quadriceps neuromuscular activation via spinal reflexes and corticospinal excitability pathways, minimizing clinical impairments of muscle weakness with disinhibitory modalities or alternate forms of training. The underlying neurophysiological impairment is treated before or in conjunction with addressing clinical impairments in step 2 before moving to further steps. Addressing the underlying neurophysiological impairments may be the catalyst for developing gains in muscle strength and functional limitations, as well as limiting patient disability.

Disinhibitory interventions are modalities used in conjunction with therapeutic exercise for the purpose of targeting specific spinal reflexive or cortical excitability pathways that contribute to neuromuscular inhibition.[29] Disinhibitory interventions can improve neuromuscular activation by stimulating receptors around the joint, which results in an altered afferent signal propagated to the central nervous system. The ultimate result of the altered afferent signal may be excitation of motor neurons innervating the previously inhibited muscle.[30] Disinhibitory interventions are not intended to be used as stand-alone therapy but rather as modalities that are typically applied before or while engaging in therapeutic exercise (**Table 1**), thus allowing patients with knee injury to perform therapeutic exercises in a state of diminished neuromuscular inhibition (see **Fig. 1**). The following sections provide evidence regarding the efficacy of specific disinhibitory interventions, along with mechanisms by which each may be used to target neuromuscular inhibition.

TRANSCUTANEOUS ELECTRICAL NERVE STIMULATION

Although traditionally used to relieve pain, transcutaneous electrical nerve stimulation (TENS) positioned over an injured joint may serve to increase neuromuscular activation of the surrounding musculature. The sensory stimuli delivered by TENS over the injured joint are hypothesized to target inhibitory presynaptic reflex mechanisms[31] that are responsible for quadriceps dysfunction.[32] TENS has been used to increase quadriceps strength in patients following ACL reconstruction[33] and patients with osteoarthritis.[34] A recent systematic review evaluating the efficacy of disinhibitory interventions for increasing voluntary quadriceps activation found that TENS produces the strongest and most consistent effects of increasing voluntary quadriceps activation compared with other disinhibitory modalities that have been studied.[29] In people with knee osteoarthritis, TENS applied to the knee produces immediate improvements in neuromuscular quadriceps activation in the first 45 minutes of TENS application.[35] Additionally, osteoarthritis subjects receiving TENS coupled with therapeutic exercise over a 4-week period demonstrate increased neuromuscular activation when compared with a group that completed the exercises protocol without the TENS.[36] Increases in neuromuscular quadriceps activation following TENS application is not associated with changes in pain, suggesting that improvement in neuromuscular quadriceps activation may occur due to disinhibitory mechanisms and not pain modulation.[35] Although TENS coupled with exercise following ACL-R increased quadriceps strength and neuromuscular activation following 2 weeks of therapy, the increases were not different than ACL-R subjects who participated in exercise alone.[33] Research is needed to determine the optimal TENS dosage needed to improve neuromuscular outcomes in patients with various knee conditions. The portability of TENS units allows this disinhibitory intervention to be easily incorporated into a rehabilitation program and patients are able to use TENS while performing rehabilitation exercises or activities of daily living.

NEUROMUSCULAR ELECTRICAL STIMULATION

Neuromuscular electrical stimulation (NMES) directly targets the inhibited muscle in an attempt to increase strength by decreasing atrophy, which differs from TENS, which targets receptors around the injured joint. NMES uses a high-intensity stimulus administered directly to the inhibited musculature to activate the inhibited α-motor neurons.[37–39] There are numerous reviews highlighting the ability of NMES for increasing quadriceps strength in patients with knee osteoarthritis[40] or total knee arthroplasty[41] and following ACL reconstruction.[42] Additionally, NMES can increase quadriceps muscle strength in adults with advanced stage diseases (COPD, chronic heart failure, and

Table 1
Pros and cons regarding the clinical use of different disinhibitory modalities for specifically addressing neuromuscular voluntary quadriceps activation in different knee pathologic states

Modality	Clinical Usefulness		Change in Neuromuscular Voluntary Quadriceps Activation in Different Knee Conditions[a]
	Pros	Cons	
Transcutaneous Electrical Nerve Stimulation	Portability, Easily used during exercise and daily life, Most disinhibitory effects, Comfortable stimulus	Some set-up required by patient	↑OA (Pietrosimone et al, 2009, 2011)
Neuromuscular Electrical Nerve Stimulation	Targets muscle atrophy	Therapeutic doses are often uncomfortable	↑TKA (Stevens et al, 2004) ↓OA (Palmieri-Smith et al, 2010)
Cryotherapy	Easily accessible, Disinhibitory affects last while body part is rewarming	Unable to use during exercise	↑OA (Pietrosimone et al, 2009) ↑Healthy (Pietrosimone et al, 2009)
Manual Therapy	No need for additional equipment	Requires advanced training for some techniques, Treatment of 1 patient at a time, Minimal effects on activation and strength	= AKP (Grindstaff et al, 2012; Drover et al, 2004; Suter et al, 1999) = Healthy (Grindstaff et al, 2009)
Transcranial Magnetic Stimulation	Moderate effect sizes indicating disinhibitory affects up to 1 h after removal of modality	High cost, Not practical to be used in most settings, Unable to use during exercise	= Partial meniscectomy (Gibbons et al, 2010)
Electromyograph Biofeedback	Provides an external feedback that targets corticospinal excitability	Requires special equipment that may be expensive and unfamiliar to clinicians	No data
Vibration	Influences many receptors in lower extremity	Treatment parameters are unclear	↑ACL-R (Brunetti et al, 2006; Fu et al, 2013; Moezy et al, 2008) ↑Artificial effusion (Blackburn et al, 2014)
	Easily used during exercise, Requires minimal training to administer, Comfortable stimulus	Whole body vibration is costly and not portable	—

Abbreviations: AKP, anterior knee pain; OA, osteoarthritis; TKA, total knee arthroplasty.
[a] Effect of activation compared with controls or baseline values before intervention was applied: ↑, increased; ↓, decreased; =, unchanged.

cancer).[43] However, there is conflicting evidence regarding how successful NMES is for improving quadriceps activation because greater improvements in quadriceps function were noted in subjects with knee arthroplasty following 6 weeks of strengthening augmented with NMES compared with strengthening alone,[44] whereas 4 weeks of NMES alone did not enhance quadriceps function in subjects with knee osteoarthritis.[45]

CRYOTHERAPY

Cryotherapy is commonly used for its analgesic benefits, yet it is also capable of disinhibiting musculature surrounding an injured joint. Cryotherapy increases neuromuscular quadriceps activation in individuals with knee osteoarthritis, as evidenced by increases in neuromuscular quadriceps activation up to 45 minutes following cryotherapy application.[35] Patients with knee osteoarthritis presented with moderate increases in voluntary quadriceps activation immediately following and 10 minutes after cryotherapy was removed from the knee. Neuromuscular activation continued to increase above that of earlier time points 25 minutes after cryotherapy had been removed.[35] This has important implications for incorporating cryotherapy into a clinical rehabilitation program. Neuromuscular benefits sustained following the removal of cryotherapy may be a function of rewarming of thermoreceptors, which alters the nature of the afferent stimuli, thereby exciting the central nervous system. Logistically, cryotherapy treatments may be cumbersome to administer during movement because it limits the ability to perform active exercises while it is actively applied. If the disinhibitory effects of cryotherapy can last for a period of time following cryotherapy removal, clinicians may be able to implement cryotherapy with therapeutic exercise. Clinicians may choose to apply cryotherapy immediately before performing exercise, thereby allowing exercise to be performed during a period of time when neuromuscular activation is high. However, there is no evidence on the long-term efficacy of augmenting traditional rehabilitation with cryotherapy.

MANUAL THERAPY

Manual therapy is used for the purpose of stimulating sensory receptors in and around a joint or to correct boney malalignments, thereby disinhibiting the musculature surrounding the joint and increasing neuromuscular activation and strength that can be produced during therapeutic exercise.[46–49] Currently, lumbopelvic manipulation is the most commonly studied manual therapy for improving neuromuscular quadriceps activation; however, this intervention has demonstrated contradictory findings.[47–49] Current evidence is contradictory because pelvic manipulation (consisting of a high-velocity low-amplitude thrust in the side-lying position) has been found to cause increased neuromuscular quadriceps activation[49] or not change neuromuscular quadriceps activation from baseline[48] in subjects with anterior knee pain. Active release technique on the quadriceps does not affect neuromuscular quadriceps activation or strength in subjects with anterior knee pain.[46] All previous manual therapy studies[46–49] have investigated time points immediately following the intervention (0, 20, 40, and 60 minutes). The strongest effects for manual therapy on improving neuromuscular quadriceps activation were observed immediately following the intervention, with negligible effect sizes being observed at 40 and 60 minutes after intervention.

TRANSCRANIAL MAGNETIC STIMULATION

Transcranial magnetic stimulation (TMS) uses an externally applied magnetic stimulus to the motor cortex to create descending contraction of a muscle in the periphery.[50] TMS can be used as a research tool to quantify excitability of the motor cortex in the brain, as well as an intervention to increase both quadriceps strength and voluntary activation in healthy participants,[51,52] subjects following total knee arthroplasty,[53] and subjects following partial meniscectomy.[54] Pervious experiments using TMS as an intervention applied a single maximal magnetic stimulus to the motor cortex while the participant performed a maximal voluntary isometric contraction. The effectiveness of disinhibitory TMS may be due to posttetanic potentiation, which creates a greater synaptic efficiency between neurons after the delivery of the TMS stimulus.[55] Further research is needed to determine which patients would benefit most from TMS and how TMS could eventually be incorporated as a clinical intervention for knee injury. The studies evaluating the effect of TMS on neuromuscular activation have not assessed its benefits past 60 minutes. Future studies should seek to determine the long-term effects of TMS on increasing neuromuscular activation.

VIBRATION

Vibratory stimuli applied to a muscle can acutely improve muscle strength, power, and activation.[56–61] Vibratory stimuli enhance muscle function via excitation of the primary muscle spindle endings (Ia afferent neuron) from rapid and repeated muscle lengthening.[62] This results in a reflexive contribution to muscle force production known as the tonic vibration reflex. Greater reflexive activity accounts for heightened muscle activity while vibration is applied but does not account for improved function following the cessation of vibration (as long as 30 minutes) observed in several studies.[61,63,64] There is some evidence that whole body vibration decreases fast-twitch motor unit recruitment thresholds[65] and facilitates corticospinal activity from the brain,[66,67] which may enhance the sustained neuromuscular effects from vibration. Vibration can be delivered indirectly (ie, whole body vibration platforms) or directly to a muscle-tendon unit. Direct muscle[57,61,68,69] and whole body[56,57,59,60,63] vibration can acutely improve muscle function and thus would be appropriate as adjunct therapies to traditional rehabilitation methods. Whole body vibration stimulates multiple receptors throughout the lower extremity, such as cutaneous receptors in the foot and mechanoreceptors in other joints,[70] which may increase afferent input to increase reflexive inhibition. Additionally, whole body vibration influences motor unit firing frequency and synchronization, muscle tuning, intramuscular coordination, and central motor command.[71] Whole body vibration and direct quadriceps muscle vibration improve quadriceps strength in patients with ACL-R.[72–74] Vibratory stimuli are commonly delivered while an individual maintains an isometric contraction or squat position. This position increases tension in the muscle and enhances signal transmission.[75] Unfortunately, treatment parameters (duration, frequency, and amplitude) are heterogeneous between studies, making a standard prescription difficult to quantify. However, extended periods of vibration may cause a reduction in muscle strength due to fatigue, neurotransmitter depletion, and presynaptic inhibition. Therefore, brief (3–5 minute) or intermittent (30–60 second) vibration exposures are most suitable to elicit an acute enhancement in muscle function.[76] The optimal frequency and amplitude for vibration treatments is unclear. However, lower limb muscles respond to stimuli similar to their natural frequency of 5 to 65 Hz.[77,78] There is some evidence to suggest that 30 Hz vibration is ideal to elicit a response in the lower extremity.[60,61,79] Amplitude is commonly expressed as peak-to-peak, and is typically between 1 and 12 mm.[76] Importantly, frequency and amplitude settings will influence the acceleration applied to the body, similar to adding extra loads in conventional resistance training.

Therefore, a high level of acceleration could be harmful. Common acceleration levels in studies reporting gains in muscle function range from 2 to 18g.[76]

BIOFEEDBACK

Biofeedback (BF) is a modality used to provide information to a patient about specific physiologic events that are often inherently difficult to perceive. In rehabilitation, feedback is commonly used to alter movements, such as landing from a jump[80] or running gait,[81] or to improve muscle activation via electromyographic BF (EMG-BF). EMG-BF involves an external focus of attention, typically with visual or auditory cues, that represents the underlying muscle activation. There is consistent evidence to suggest that motor learning[82] and retention is improved as the focus of attention is transitioned from an internal emphasis (eg, instructing a patient to contract muscles with maximal effort) to an external emphasis (eg, instructing a patient to manipulate a bar graph that represents underlying muscle activation). There is little evidence that augmenting resistance training with EMG-BF for the purpose of improving muscle activation will benefit strength development in healthy participants.[83] A recent systematic review found that individuals with anterior knee pain or knee osteoarthritis receive the greatest quadriceps strength improvements from EMG-BF compared with improvements found in healthy participants.[83] One explanation for the improved strength following the use of EMG-BF is improved descending excitability from pathways associated with excitability of the primary motor cortex. Therefore, EMG-BF may be a viable modality that can specifically be integrated into therapeutic rehabilitation programs for patients that have cortical excitability deficits.

ELICITING STRENGTH GAINS WITH DIFFERENT TYPES OF NEUROMUSCULAR TRAINING

In addition to using disinhibitory modalities with therapeutic exercises to elicit greater neuromuscular activation, different types of training may be able to influence neural drive to musculature for the purpose of maximizing muscle strength.

ECCENTRIC TRAINING

Traditional rehabilitation following joint injury focuses on improving muscle strength through concentric muscle activity in which the force produced by the muscle is greater than the external force and shortening of the muscle occurs. During eccentric muscle contraction, an external force exceeds the force exerted by the muscle, which results in muscle lengthening during muscle contraction.[84] Additionally, neural activity from the motor cortex occurs sooner and is stronger during eccentric muscle contractions than during concentric contractions.[85] Eccentric exercise training improves strength in subjects following ACL-R[86–90] and in those with knee osteoarthritis[91] compared with the same subject cohorts who have participated in concentric exercise training. Clinicians should only use eccentric training to increase neural drive to the muscle when healing of injured tissue will allow eccentric exercises to be implemented safely without risk of further injury.

HIGH-VELOCITY TRAINING

In both healthy[92–94] and pathologic populations,[95,96] muscle power has been demonstrated be an important neuromuscular factor associated with physical function. Although a diminished capacity to generate muscle power occurs due to normal aging,[97] decreased muscular power may be exacerbated in older patients who also have knee osteoarthritis, resulting in loss of further physical function and mobility.[98]

High-velocity training, or training patients to focus on moving weight with increased speeds of contraction, has been hypothesized to be a catalyst for neural adaptations that may increase muscle performance related to power, without eliciting hypertrophic muscular changes.[99] High-velocity training has been successfully implemented in older adults with osteoarthritis in an attempt to improve muscle strength as well as functional performance.[98,100–102] Fukumoto and colleagues[100] compared 8 weeks of a home-based resistance training program using either high-velocity or low-velocity muscle contractions in women with hip osteoarthritis. The Timed Up and Go was significantly improved in the high-velocity training group compared with the low-velocity training group.[100] Sayers and colleagues[102] found no difference in strength but did find power improvements in subjects with knee osteoarthritis following 12 weeks of either high-velocity or low-velocity training on pneumatic leg press and knee extension machines. The investigators concluded that the high-velocity training produced a broader training effect with regards to peak power compared with the low-velocity training group across a range of resistance that is typically experienced in activities of daily life.[102] Clinicians may need to use caution regarding the stage of rehabilitation in which high-velocity training is implemented following knee injury. Every knee injury incorporates different pathophysiology and, therefore, requires variable healing times. Before using high-velocity training, clinicians should ensure that any injured or surgically repaired tissue has sufficiently healed to withstand the exercise.

HIGH-INTENSITY TRAINING

It has been suggested weight-training loads applied during traditional strength training may be inadequate for producing satisfactory improvements in muscle strength.[103] High-intensity training (HIT), or heavy resistance training, is performed with high-resistance loads that are close to maximal intensity. Andersen and colleagues[104] demonstrated that heavy resistance exercises increased neuromuscular activation compared with conventional rehabilitation exercises. Bieler and colleagues[105] reported that maximal muscle power was regained in ACL-R subjects who performed the HIT compared with the low-intensity exercise group. High-intensity resistance training has also been implemented in patients with knee osteoarthritis.[106–108] Subjects with knee osteoarthritis demonstrated improvements in strength following 6-month[106] and 12-month HIT interventions[107]; whereas McQuade and colleagues[108] did not report changes in muscle strength following HIT. Future research is needed to determine which patients with knee injury would benefit most from HIT and how to best implement HIT in the clinic. Similar to high-velocity training, clinicians should ensure that the strength of the healing tissue around the joint can withstand HIT. Additionally, clinicians should ensure that proper movement patterns are maintained during HIT, thereby minimizing aberrant compensatory movements that may lead to future musculoskeletal injury.

SUMMARY

Muscle strength plays a strong role in the maintaining physical function in patients who have various knee injuries or osteoarthritis. Targeting neuromuscular activation deficits that are associated with the loss of muscle strength following injury may be critical for (1) minimizing the risk for developing persistent strength deficits following acute injury and (2) providing a novel clinical breakthrough therapy technique for patients who have developed persistent muscle weakness long after acute knee injury or in conjunction with chronic knee condition. Disinhibitory interventions described in this article (eg, TENS, cryotherapy, vibration) are designed to augment traditional thera-peutic exercise for the purpose of allowing more neuromuscular activation during ther-apeutic exercise and resulting in more substantial gains in strength. Targeting neuromuscular activation with disinhibitory modalities may be most beneficial for pa-tients who do not respond to traditional knee injury rehabilitation, or who do not develop adequate strength from therapeutic exercise alone. In addition to using dis-inhibitory modalities with traditional strength training, other types of training (eg, eccentric strengthening, high-velocity training, and HIT) can be implemented to further increase neural drive during exercise.

REFERENCES

1. Kojima N, Kim H, Saito K, et al. Association of knee-extension strength with instrumental activities of daily living in community-dwelling older adults. Geriatr Gerontol Int 2014;14(3):674–80.
2. Hart J, Pietrosimone B, Hertel J, et al. Quadriceps activation failure following knee injuries: a systematic review. J Athl Train 2010;45(1):87–97.
3. Pietrosimone BG, Lepley AS, Ericksen HM, et al. Quadriceps strength and cor-ticospinal excitability as predictors of disability after anterior cruciate ligament reconstruction. J Sport Rehabil 2013;22(1):1–6.
4. McLeod MM, Gribble P, Pfile KR, et al. Effects of arthroscopic partial meniscec-tomy on quadriceps strength: a systematic review. J Sport Rehabil 2012;21(3): 285–95.
5. Hart J, Ko J, Konold T, et al. Sagittal plane knee joint moments following anterior cruciate ligament injury and reconstruction: a systematic review. Clin Biomech (Bristol, Avon) 2010;25(4):277–83.
6. Gardinier E, Manal K, Buchanan T, et al. Gait and neuromuscular asymmetries after acute anterior cruciate ligament rupture. Med Sci Sports Exerc 2012; 44(8):1490–6.
7. Noehren BW, Miller C, Lattermann C. Long-term gait deviations in anterior cru-ciate ligament-reconstructed females. Med Sci Sports Exerc 2013;45(7): 1340–7.
8. Shabani B, Bytyqi D, Lustig S, et al. Gait changes of the ACL-deficient knee 3D kinematic assessment. Knee Surg Sports Traumatol Arthrosc 2014. PMID: 25026934 [Epub ahead of print].
9. Scanlan S, Donahue J, Andriacchi T. The in vivo relationship between anterior neutral tibial position and loss of knee extension after transtibial ACL reconstruc-tion. Knee 2013;46(5):849–54.
10. Palmieri-Smith R, Thomas A. A neuromuscular mechanism of posttraumatic osteoarthritis associated with ACL injury. Exerc Sport Sci Rev 2009;37(3): 147–53.
11. Radin E, Martin R, Burr D, et al. Effects of mechanical loading on the tissues of the rabbit knee. J Orthop Res 1984;2(3):221–34.
12. Han S, Seerattan R, Herzog W. Mechanical loading of in situ chondrocytes in lapine retropatellar cartilage after anterior cruciate ligament transection. J R Soc Interface 2010;7(47):895–903.
13. Hunt M, Hinman R, Metcalf B, et al. Quadriceps strength is not related to gait impact loading in knee osteoarthritis. Knee 2010;17(4):296–302.
14. Luc B, Gribble P, Pietrosimone B. Osteoarthritis prevalence following anterior cruciate ligament reconstruction: a systematic review and numbers needed to treat analysis. J Athl Train 2014;49(6):806–19.

15. Seymour JM, Spruit MA, Hopkinson NS, et al. The prevalence of quadriceps weakness in COPD and the relationship with disease severity. Eur Respir J 2010;36(1):81–8.
16. Shrikrishna D, Patel M, Tanner RJ, et al. Quadriceps wasting and physical inactivity in patients with COPD. Eur Respir J 2012;40(5):1115–22.
17. Kamiya K, Mezzani A, Hotta K, et al. Quadriceps isometric strength as a predictor of exercise capacity in coronary artery disease patients. Eur J Prev Cardiol 2014;21(10):1285–91.
18. Kalyani RR, Tra Y, Yeh HC, et al. Quadriceps strength, quadriceps power, and gait speed in older U.S. adults with diabetes mellitus: results from the National Health and Nutrition Examination Survey, 1999–2002. J Am Geriatr Soc 2013; 61(5):769–75.
19. Swallow E, Reyes E, Hopkinson N, et al. Quadriceps strength predicts mortality in patients with moderate to severe chronic obstructive pulmonary disease. Thorax 2007;62(2):115–20.
20. Nuesch E, Dieppe P, Reichenbach S, et al. All cause and disease specific mortality in patients with knee or hip osteoarthritis: population based cohort study. BMJ 2011;342:d1165.
21. Fitzgerald GK, Piva SR, Irrgang JJ, et al. Quadriceps activation failure as a moderator of the relationship between quadriceps strength and physical function in individuals with knee osteoarthritis. Arthritis Rheum 2004;51(1):40–8.
22. Pietrosimone B, Thomas A, Saliba S, et al. Association between quadriceps strength and self-reported physical activity in people with knee osteoarthritis. Int J Sports Phys Ther 2014;9(3):320–8.
23. Hurley MV, Jones DW, Newham DJ. Arthrogenic quadriceps inhibition and rehabilitation of patients with extensive traumatic knee injuries. Clin Sci (Lond) 1994; 86(3):305–10.
24. Mikesky AE, Mazzuca SA, Brandt KD, et al. Effects of strength training on the incidence and progression of knee osteoarthritis. Arthritis Rheum 2006;55(5): 690–9.
25. Hopkins JT, Ingersoll C. Arthrogenic muscle inhibition: a limiting factor in joint rehabilitation. J Sport Rehabil 2000;9(2):135–59.
26. Heroux M, Tremblay F. Corticomotor excitability associated with unilateral knee dysfunction secondary to anterior cruciate ligament injury. Knee Surg Sports Traumatol Arthrosc 2006;14:823–33.
27. Pietrosimone B, Lepley A, Ericksen H, et al. Spinal reflexive and corticomotor excitability alterations following anterior cruciate ligament reconstruction. J Athl Train, in press. http://dx.doi.org/10.4085/1062-6050-50.1.11.
28. Pietrosimone B, Saliba S. Changes in voluntary quadriceps activation predict changes in quadriceps strength after therapeutic exercise in patients with knee osteoarthritis. Knee 2012;19(6):939–43.
29. Harkey MS, Gribble PA, Pietrosimone BG. Disinhibitory interventions and voluntary quadriceps activation: a systematic review. J Athl Train 2014;49(3):411–21.
30. Pietrosimone BG, Hopkins JT, Ingersoll CD. The role of disinhibitory modalities in joint injury rehabilitation. Athl Ther Today 2008;13(6):2–5.
31. Iles JF. Evidence for cutaneous and corticospinal modulation of presynaptic inhibition of Ia afferents from the human lower limb. J Physiol 1996;491(1): 197–207.
32. Palmieri RM, Tom JA, Edwards JE, et al. Arthrogenic muscle response induced by an experimental knee joint effusion is mediated by pre- and post-synaptic spinal mechanisms. J Electromyogr Kinesiol 2004;14(6):631–40.

33. Hart JM, Kuenze CM, Pietrosimone BG, et al. Quadriceps function in anterior cruciate ligament-deficient knees exercising with transcutaneous electrical nerve stimulation and cryotherapy: a randomized controlled study. Clin Rehabil 2012;26(11):974–81.

34. Cherian JJ, Kapadia BH, Bhave A, et al. Use of transcutaneous electrical nerve stimulation device in early osteoarthritis of the knee. J Knee Surg 2014. PMID: 25162407 [Epub ahead of print].

35. Pietrosimone BG, Hart JM, Saliba SA, et al. Immediate effects of transcutaneous electrical nerve stimulation and focal knee joint cooling on quadriceps activation. Med Sci Sports Exerc 2009;41(6):1175–81.

36. Pietrosimone BG, Saliba SA, Hart JM, et al. Effects of transcutaneous electrical nerve stimulation and therapeutic exercise on quadriceps activation in people with tibiofemoral osteoarthritis. J Orthop Sports Phys Ther 2011;41(1):4–12.

37. Fitzgerald GK, Piva SR, Irrgang JJ. A modified neuromuscular electrical stimulation protocol for quadriceps strength training following anterior cruciate ligament reconstruction. J Orthop Sports Phys Ther 2003;33(9):492–501.

38. Snyder-Mackler L, Delitto A, Bailey SL, et al. Strength of the quadriceps femoris muscle and functional recovery after reconstruction of the anterior cruciate ligament. A prospective, randomized clinical trial of electrical stimulation. J Bone Joint Surg Am 1995;77(8):1166–73.

39. Snyder-Mackler L, Ladin Z, Schepsis AA, et al. Electrical stimulation of the thigh muscles after reconstruction of the anterior cruciate ligament. Effects of electrically elicited contraction of the quadriceps femoris and hamstring muscles on gait and on strength of the thigh muscles. J Bone Joint Surg Am 1991;73(7): 1025–36.

40. de Oliveira Melo M, Aragao FA, Vaz MA. Neuromuscular electrical stimulation for muscle strengthening in elderly with knee osteoarthritis - a systematic review. Complement Ther Clin Pract 2013;19(1):27–31.

41. Kittelson AJ, Stackhouse SK, Stevens-Lapsley JE. Neuromuscular electrical stimulation after total joint arthroplasty: a critical review of recent controlled studies. Eur J Phys Rehabil Med 2013;49(6):909–20.

42. Kim KM, Croy T, Hertel J, et al. Effects of neuromuscular electrical stimulation after anterior cruciate ligament reconstruction on quadriceps strength, function, and patient-oriented outcomes: a systematic review. J Orthop Sports Phys Ther 2010;40(7):383–91.

43. Maddocks M, Gao W, Higginson IJ, et al. Neuromuscular electrical stimulation for muscle weakness in adults with advanced disease. Cochrane Database Syst Rev 2013;(1):CD009419.

44. Stevens JE, Mizner RL, Snyder-Mackler L. Neuromuscular electrical stimulation for quadriceps muscle strengthening after bilateral total knee arthroplasty: a case series. J Orthop Sports Phys Ther 2004;34(1):21–9.

45. Palmieri-Smith RM, Thomas AC, Karvonen-Gutierrez C, et al. A clinical trial of neuromuscular electrical stimulation in improving quadriceps muscle strength and activation among women with mild and moderate osteoarthritis. Phys Ther 2010;90(10):1441–52.

46. Drover JM, Forand DR, Herzog W. Influence of active release technique on quadriceps inhibition and strength: a pilot study. J Manipulative Physiol Ther 2004;27(6):408–13.

47. Grindstaff TL, Hertel J, Beazell JR, et al. Effects of lumbopelvic joint manipulation on quadriceps activation and strength in healthy individuals. Man Ther 2009;14(4):415–20.

48. Grindstaff TL, Hertel J, Beazell JR, et al. Lumbopelvic joint manipulation and quadriceps activation of people with patellofemoral pain syndrome. J Athl Train 2012;47(1):24–31.
49. Suter E, McMorland G, Herzog W, et al. Decrease in quadriceps inhibition after sacroiliac joint manipulation in patients with anterior knee pain. J Manipulative Physiol Ther 1999;22(3):149–53.
50. Anand S, Hotson J. Transcranial magnetic stimulation: neurophysiological applications and safety. Brain Cogn 2002;50(3):366–86.
51. Urbach D, Awiszus F. Effects of transcranial magnetic stimulation on results of the twitch interpolation technique. Muscle Nerve 2000;23(7):1125–8.
52. Urbach D, Awiszus F. Stimulus strength related effect of transcranial magnetic stimulation on maximal voluntary contraction force of human quadriceps femoris muscle. Exp Brain Res 2002;142(1):25–31.
53. Urbach D, Berth A, Awiszus F. Effect of transcranial magnetic stimulation on voluntary activation in patients with quadriceps weakness. Muscle Nerve 2005;32(2):164–9.
54. Gibbons CE, Pietrosimone BG, Hart JM, et al. Transcranial magnetic stimulation and volitional quadriceps activation. J Athl Train 2010;45(6):570–9.
55. Purves D, Augustine G, Fitzpatrick D, et al. Neuroscience. 2nd edition. Sunderland (MA): Sinauer Associates; 2001.
56. Abercromby AF, Amonette WE, Layne CS, et al. Vibration exposure and biodynamic responses during whole-body vibration training. Med Sci Sports Exerc 2007;39(10):1794–800.
57. Blackburn JT, Pamukoff DN, Sakr M, et al. Whole body and local muscle vibration reduce artificially induced quadriceps arthrogenic inhibition. Arch Phys Med Rehabil 2014;95(11):2021–8.
58. Bosco C, Cardinale M, Tsarpela O. Influence of vibration on mechanical power and electromyogram activity in human arm flexor muscles. Eur J Appl Physiol Occup Physiol 1999;79(4):306–11.
59. Bosco C, Colli R, Introini E, et al. Adaptive responses of human skeletal muscle to vibration exposure. Clin Physiol 1999;19(2):183–7.
60. Cardinale M, Lim J. Electromyography activity of vastus lateralis muscle during whole-body vibrations of different frequencies. J Strength Cond Res 2003;17(3): 621–4.
61. Pamukoff DN, Ryan ED, Troy Blackburn J. The acute effects of local muscle vibration frequency on peak torque, rate of torque development, and EMG activity. J Electromyogr Kinesiol 2014;24(6):888–94.
62. Eklund G, Hagbarth KE. Normal variability of tonic vibration reflexes in man. Exp Neurol 1966;16(1):80–92.
63. Bazett-Jones DM, Finch HW, Dugan EL. Comparing the effects of various whole-body vibration accelerations on counter-movement jump performance. J Sports Sci Med 2008;7(1):144–50.
64. McBride JM, Nuzzo JL, Dayne AM, et al. Effect of an acute bout of whole body vibration exercise on muscle force output and motor neuron excitability. J Strength Cond Res 2010;24(1):184–9.
65. Pollock RD, Woledge RC, Martin FC, et al. Effects of whole body vibration on motor unit recruitment and threshold. J Appl Physiol (1985) 2012;112(3): 388–95.
66. Mileva KN, Bowtell JL, Kossev AR. Effects of low-frequency whole-body vibration on motor-evoked potentials in healthy men. Exp Physiol 2009;94(1): 103–16.

67. Siggelkow S, Kossev A, Schubert M, et al. Modulation of motor evoked potentials by muscle vibration: the role of vibration frequency. Muscle Nerve 1999; 22(11):1544–8.

68. Couto BP, Silva HR, Filho AG, et al. Acute effects of resistance training with local vibration. Int J Sports Med 2013;34(9):814–9.

69. Ribot-Ciscar E, Butler JE, Thomas CK. Facilitation of triceps brachii muscle contraction by tendon vibration after chronic cervical spinal cord injury. J Appl Physiol (1985) 2003;94(6):2358–67.

70. Pollock RD, Provan S, Martin FC, et al. The effects of whole body vibration on balance, joint position sense and cutaneous sensation. Eur J Appl Physiol 2011;111(12):3069–77.

71. Cochrane DJ. The potential neural mechanisms of acute indirect vibration. J Sports Sci Med 2011;10(1):19–30.

72. Moezy A, Olyaei G, Hadian M, et al. A comparative study of whole body vibration training and conventional training on knee proprioception and postural stability after anterior cruciate ligament reconstruction. Br J Sports Med 2008;42(5): 373–8.

73. Brunetti O, Filippi GM, Lorenzini M, et al. Improvement of posture stability by vibratory stimulation following anterior cruciate ligament reconstruction. Knee Surg Sports Traumatol Arthrosc 2006;14(11):1180–7.

74. Fu CL, Yung SH, Law KY, et al. The effect of early whole-body vibration therapy on neuromuscular control after anterior cruciate ligament reconstruction: a randomized controlled trial. Am J Sports Med 2013;41(4):804–14.

75. Burke D, Gandevia SC. The human muscle spindle and its fusimotor control. Neural Control of Movement 1995;19–25.

76. Cochrane DJ. Vibration exercise: the potential benefits. Int J Sports Med 2011; 32(2):75–99.

77. Wakeling JM, Nigg BM. Soft-tissue vibrations in the quadriceps measured with skin mounted transducers. J Biomech 2001;34(4):539–43.

78. Wakeling JM, Nigg BM. Modification of soft tissue vibrations in the leg by muscular activity. J Appl Physiol (1985) 2001;90(2):412–20.

79. Da Silva ME, Nunez VM, Vaamonde D, et al. Effects of different frequencies of whole body vibration on muscular performance. Biol Sport 2006;23(3):267–82.

80. Ericksen H, Gribble P, Pfile K, et al. Different modes of feedback and peak vertical ground reaction force during jump landing: a systematic review. J Athl Train 2013;48(5):685–95.

81. Crowell H, Milner C, Hamill J, et al. Reducing impact loading during running with the use of real-time visual feedback. J Orthop Sports Phys Ther 2010;40(4):206–13.

82. McNevin N, Shea C, Wulf G. Increasing the distance of an external focus of attention enhances learning. Phychol Res 2003;67:22–9.

83. Lepley A, Gribble P, Pietrosimone B. Effects of electromyographic biofeedback on quadriceps strength: a systematic review. J Strength Cond Res 2012;26(3): 873–82.

84. Lindstedt SL, LaStayo PC, Reich TE. When active muscles lengthen: properties and consequences of eccentric contractions. News Physiol Sci 2001;16:256–61.

85. Fang Y, Siemionow V, Sahgal V, et al. Distinct brain activation patterns for human maximal voluntary eccentric and concentric muscle actions. Brain 2004; 1023(2):200–12.

86. Brasileiro JS, Pinto OM, Avila MA, et al. Functional and morphological changes in the quadriceps muscle induced by eccentric training after ACL reconstruction. Rev Bras Fisioter 2011;15(4):284–90.

87. Coury HJ, Brasileiro JS, Salvini TF, et al. Change in knee kinematics during gait after eccentric isokinetic training for quadriceps in subjects submitted to anterior cruciate ligament reconstruction. Gait Posture 2006;24(3):370–4.
88. Gerber JP, Marcus RL, Dibble LE, et al. Effects of early progressive eccentric exercise on muscle structure after anterior cruciate ligament reconstruction. J Bone Joint Surg Am 2007;89(3):559–70.
89. Gerber JP, Marcus RL, Dibble LE, et al. Effects of early progressive eccentric exercise on muscle size and function after anterior cruciate ligament reconstruction: a 1-year follow-up study of a randomized clinical trial. Phys Ther 2009; 89(1):51–9.
90. Kinikli GI, Yuksel I, Baltaci G, et al. The effect of progressive eccentric and concentric training on functional performance after autogenous hamstring anterior cruciate ligament reconstruction: a randomized controlled study. Acta Orthop Traumatol Turc 2014;48(3):283–9.
91. Gur H, Cakin N, Akova B, et al. Concentric versus combined concentric-eccentric isokinetic training: effects on functional capacity and symptoms in patients with osteoarthrosis of the knee. Arch Phys Med Rehabil 2002;83(3): 308–16.
92. Sayers SP, Guralnik JM, Thombs LA, et al. Effect of leg muscle contraction velocity on functional performance in older men and women. J Am Geriatr Soc 2005;53(3):467–71.
93. Bean JF, Kiely DK, Herman S, et al. The relationship between leg power and physical performance in mobility-limited older people. J Am Geriatr Soc 2002; 50(3):461–7.
94. Foldvari M, Clark M, Laviolette LC, et al. Association of muscle power with functional status in community-dwelling elderly women. J Gerontol A Biol Sci Med Sci 2000;55(4):M192–9.
95. Hsieh CJ, Indelicato PA, Moser MW, et al. Speed, not magnitude, of knee extensor torque production is associated with self-reported knee function early after anterior cruciate ligament reconstruction. Knee Surg Sports Traumatol Arthrosc 2014. PMID: 25026933 [Epub ahead of print].
96. Berger MJ, McKenzie CA, Chess DG, et al. Quadriceps neuromuscular function and self-reported functional ability in knee osteoarthritis. J Appl Physiol (1985) 2012;113(2):255–62.
97. Skelton DA, Greig CA, Davies JM, et al. Strength, power and related functional ability of healthy people aged 65–89 years. Age Aging 1994;23(5):371–7.
98. Segal NA, Wallace R. Tolerance of an aquatic power training program by older adults with symptomatic knee osteoarthritis. Arthritis 2012;2012:895495.
99. Behm DG, Sale DG. Intended rather than actual movement velocity determines velocity-specific training response. J Appl Physiol (1985) 1993;74(1): 359–68.
100. Fukumoto Y, Tateuchi H, Ikezoe T, et al. Effects of high-velocity resistance training on muscle function, muscle properties, and physical performance in individuals with hip osteoarthritis: a randomized controlled trial. Clin Rehabil 2014; 28(1):48–58.
101. Pelletier D, Gingras-Hill C, Boissy P. Power training in patients with knee osteoarthritis: a pilot study on feasibility and efficacy. Physiother Can 2013;65(2): 176–82.
102. Sayers SP, Gibson K, Cook CR. Effect of high-speed power training on muscle performance, function, and pain in older adults with knee osteoarthritis: a pilot investigation. Arthritis Care Res (Hoboken) 2012;64(1):46–53.

103. Thomee R, Kaplan Y, Kvist J, et al. Muscle strength and hop performance criteria prior to return to sports after ACL reconstruction. Knee Surg Sports Traumatol Arthrosc 2011;19(11):1798–805.

104. Andersen LL, Magnusson SP, Nielsen M, et al. Neuromuscular activation in conventional therapeutic exercises and heavy resistance exercises: implications for rehabilitation. Phys Ther 2006;86(5):683–97.

105. Bieler T, Sobol NA, Andersen LL, et al. The effects of high-intensity versus low-intensity resistance training on leg extensor power and recovery of knee function after ACL-reconstruction. Biomed Res Int 2014;2014:278512.

106. Foroughi N, Smith RM, Lange AK, et al. Progressive resistance training and dynamic alignment in osteoarthritis: a single-blind randomised controlled trial. Clin Biomech (Bristol, Avon) 2011;26(1):71–7.

107. King LK, Birmingham TB, Kean CO, et al. Resistance training for medial compartment knee osteoarthritis and malalignment. Med Sci Sports Exerc 2008;40(8):1376–84.

108. McQuade KJ, de Oliveira AS. Effects of progressive resistance strength training on knee biomechanics during single leg step-up in persons with mild knee osteoarthritis. Clin Biomech (Bristol, Avon) 2011;26(7):741–8.

Controversies in Knee Rehabilitation

Anterior Cruciate Ligament Injury

Mathew J. Failla, PT, MSPT, SCS[a],*, Amelia J.H. Arundale, PT, DPT, SCS[a],
David S. Logerstedt, PT, PhD, SCS[a,b], Lynn Snyder-Mackler, PT, ScD, SCS[a,c]

KEYWORDS

- Anterior cruciate ligament • Knee • ACLR • ACL • Physical therapy • Athletes
- Sports physical therapy

KEY POINTS

- Undergoing anterior cruciate ligament (ACL) reconstruction does not guarantee athletes will return to their preinjury sport, and return to the preinjury competitive level of sport is unlikely.
- The risk of a second ACL injury is high in young athletes returning to sport, especially in the near term.
- The risk for developing osteoarthritis after ACL injury is high in the long term regardless of surgical intervention, and even higher if a revision procedure is required.
- Despite common misconceptions, nonoperatively managed athletes can return to sport without the need for reconstruction.
- Without differences in outcomes between early reconstruction, delayed reconstruction, and nonoperative management, counseling should start by considering nonoperative management.

INTRODUCTION

More than 250,000 anterior cruciate ligament (ACL) injuries occur yearly in the United States,[1] with 125,000 to 175,000 undergoing ACL reconstruction (ACLR).[2,3] Although standard of practice in the United States is early reconstruction for active individuals with the promise of returning to preactivity injury levels,[4,5] evidence suggests athletes are counseled that reconstruction is not required to return to high-level activity after a program of intensive neuromuscular training.[6] Others advocate counseling for a

Disclosures: None.
[a] Biomechanics and Movement Science, University of Delaware, Newark, DE, USA;
[b] Department of Physical Therapy, University of the Sciences in Philadelphia, Philadelphia, Pennsylvania; [c] Department of Physical Therapy, University of Delaware, Newark, DE, USA
* Corresponding author.
E-mail address: mfailla@udel.edu

Clin Sports Med 34 (2015) 301–312
http://dx.doi.org/10.1016/j.csm.2014.12.008
0278-5919/15/$ – see front matter © 2015 Elsevier Inc. All rights reserved.

delayed reconstruction approach[7]; however, no differences in outcomes exist between delayed and early ACLR.[6] Furthermore, athletes in the United States are commonly counseled to undergo early ACLR[5] with the promise of restoring static joint stability, minimizing further damage to the meniscii and articular cartilage,[4,8] and preserving knee joint health[5]; however, not all athletes are able to return to sport or exhibit normal knee function following reconstruction.[9] Several factors, such as impaired functional performance, knee instability and pain, reduced range of motion, quadriceps strength deficits, neuromuscular dysfunction, and biomechanical maladaptations, may account for highly variable degrees of success.

To identify the minimum set of outcomes that identifies success after ACL injury or ACLR, Lynch and colleagues[10] established consensus criteria from 1779 sports medicine professionals concerning successful outcomes after ACL injury and reconstruction. The consensus of successful outcomes were identified as no reinjury or recurrent giving way, no joint effusion, quadriceps strength symmetry, restored activity level and function, and returning to preinjury sports (**Table 1**).[10] Using these criteria, the success rates of current management after ACL injury are reviewed and recommendations are provided for the counseling of athletes after ACL injury.

IMPAIRMENT RESOLUTION

Following ACL injury or reconstruction, athletes undergo an extensive period of vigorous rehabilitation targeting functional impairments. These targeted rehabilitation protocols strive for full symmetric range of motion, adequate quadriceps strength, walking and running without frank aberrant movement, and a quiet knee: little to no joint effusion or pain.[10] Despite targeted postoperative rehabilitation, athletes commonly experience quadriceps strength deficits,[11–13] lower self-reported knee function,[14] and movement asymmetry[15,16] up to 2 years after reconstruction. The importance of quadriceps strength as a dynamic knee stabilizer has been established, because deficits have been linked to lower functional outcomes.[12,17] In a systematic review of quadriceps strength after ACLR, quadriceps strength deficits can exceed 20% 6 months after reconstruction, with deficits having the potential to persist for 2 years after reconstruction.[13] Otzel and colleagues[18] reported a 6% to 9% quadriceps deficit 3 years after reconstruction, concluding that long-term deficits after surgery were the result of lower neural drive because quadriceps atrophy measured by thigh circumference was not significantly different between limbs. Grindem and colleagues[19] reported at 2-year follow-up that 23% of nonoperatively managed athletes

Table 1		
Consensus criteria on successful outcomes after anterior cruciate ligament injury and reconstruction from 1779 sports medicine professionals		
Criterion	2 y After Operative Management (Consensus %)	2 y After Nonoperative Management (Consensus %)
Absence of giving way	96.4	96.5
Return to sports	92.4	92.7
Quadriceps strength symmetry	90.3	90.7
Absence of joint effusion	84.1	85.0
Patient-reported outcomes	83.2	83.5

Data from Lynch AD, Logerstedt DS, Grindem H, et al. Consensus criteria for defining "successful outcome" after ACL injury and reconstruction: a Delaware-Oslo ACL cohort investigation. Br J Sports Med 2013:1–9.

had greater than 10% strength deficits compared with one-third of athletes who underwent reconstruction. Another study comparing operatively and nonoperatively managed patients 2 to 5 years after ACL injury found no differences in quadriceps strength between groups, concluding that reconstructive surgery is not a prerequisite for restoring muscle function.[20] Regardless of operative or nonoperative management, quadriceps strength deficits are ubiquitous after ACL injury and can persist for the long term. The current evidence does not support ACLR as a means of improved quadriceps strength outcomes over nonoperative management after ACL injury.

OUTCOMES

Individuals do not respond uniformly to an acute ACL injury, and outcomes can vary. Most individuals decrease their activity level after ACL injury.[20–25] Although a large majority of individuals rate their knee function below normal ranges after an ACL injury, which is a common finding early after an injury,[26–30] some individuals exhibit higher perceived knee function than others early after ACL injury,[28–30] highlighting the variability in outcomes seen after ACL injury.

Knee outcome scores are lowest early after surgery and improve up to 6 years after surgery.[29,31,32] Using the Cincinnati Knee Rating System, scores improved from 60.5/100 at 12 weeks after reconstruction to 85.9/100 at 1-year follow-up.[32] By 6 months after surgery, almost half of the individuals scored greater than 90% on the Knee Outcomes Survey–Activities of Daily Living Scale (KOS-ADLS) and Global Rating Scale of Perceived Function (GRS), and 78% achieved these scores by 12 months.[14] Using the GRS, scores improved from 63.1/100 taken at week 12 to 83.3/100 at week 52.[32] Moksnes and Risberg[29] reported similar postsurgical GRS results of 86.0/100 at 1-year follow-up. Poor self-report on outcome measures after ACLR are associated with chondral injury, previous surgery, return to sport, and poor radiological grade in ipsilateral medial compartment.[33] ACLR revision and extension deficits at 3 months are also predictors of poor long-term outcomes.[34,35]

Patient-reported outcomes from multiple large surgical registries are available concerning patients after ACLR. A study from the Multicenter Orthopaedic Outcomes Network (MOON) consortium of 446 patients reported International Knee Documentation Committee Subjective Knee Form 2000 (IKDC) for patients 2 and 6 years after reconstruction.[36] The median IKDC score was 45 at baseline, increased to 75 at 2-year follow-up, and reached 77 at 6 years after reconstruction.[36] Grindem and colleagues[19] compared IKDC scores between athletes managed nonoperatively or with reconstruction at baseline and at 2 years. The nonoperative group improved from a score of 73 at baseline to a score of 89 at 2 years after injury.[19] The reconstructed group improved from 69 at baseline to 89 2 years after surgery.[19] There were no significant differences between groups at baseline or at 2-year follow-up.[19] Using the Knee Injury and Osteoarthritis Outcome Score, Frobell and colleagues[37] compared patient-reported outcomes at 5 years after ACL injury and found no significant differences in change of score from baseline to 5 years in those managed with early reconstruction versus those managed nonoperatively or with delayed reconstruction. Outcomes after ACL injury, whether managed nonoperatively or with ACLR, have similar patient-reported outcomes scores at up to 5 years after injury.

LONG-TERM JOINT HEALTH

Preventing further intra-articular injury and preserving joint surfaces for long-term knee health are purposed reasons to surgically stabilize an unstable knee.[5] Patients who had increased knee laxity after an ACL injury are more likely to have late meniscal surgery,[33] and time from ACL injury is associated with the number of chondral injuries and severity of chondral lesions.[38] Injury to menisci or articular cartilage places the knee at increased risk for the development of osteoarthritis.[39] Barenius and colleagues[39] found a 3-fold increase in knee osteoarthritis prevalence in surgically reconstructed knees 14 years after surgery. They concluded that although ACLR did not prevent secondary osteoarthritis, initial meniscal resection was a risk factor for osteoarthritis with no differences in osteoarthritis prevalence seen between graft types.[39] A recent systematic review compared operatively and nonoperatively treated patients at a mean of 14 years after ACL injury[40] and found no significant differences between groups in radiographic osteoarthritis.[40] The operative group had less subsequent surgery and meniscal tears as well as increased Tegner change scores; however, there were no differences in Lysholm or IKDC scores between groups.[40] The current evidence does not support the use of ACLR to reduce secondary knee osteoarthritis after ACL injury.

RETURN TO PREINJURY SPORTS

Returning to sports is often cited as the goals of athletes and health care professionals after ACL injury or ACLR. When asked, 90% of National Football League (NFL) head team physicians thought that 90% to 100% of NFL players returned to play after ACLR.[41] Shah and colleagues[42] found that, regardless of position, 63% of NFL athletes seen at their facility returned to play. A recent systematic review reported 81% of athletes return to any sports at all, but only 65% returned to their preinjury level, and an even smaller percentage, 55%, return to competitive sports (**Fig. 1**).[43] This review found that younger athletes, men, and elite athletes were more likely to return to sports.[43] Similar reports within this range are common when examining amateur athletes by sport. McCullough and colleagues[44] report that 63% of high school and 69% of college football players return to sport. Shelbourne and colleagues[45] found that 97% of high school basketball players return to play, 93% of high school women soccer players, and 80% of high school male soccer players returned to play. Brophy and colleagues[46] found a slightly different trend in soccer players: 72% returned to play, whereas 61% returned to the same level of competition, but when broken down by

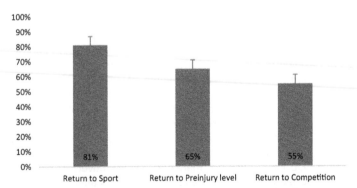

Fig. 1. Reported return-to-sport rates after ACLR from Arden and colleagues' 2014 systematic review and meta-analysis. (*Data from* Ardern CL, Taylor NF, Feller JA, et al. Fifty-five per cent return to competitive sport following anterior cruciate ligament reconstruction surgery: an updated systematic review and meta-analysis including aspects of physical functioning and contextual factors. Br J Sports Med 2014;48:1543–52.)

sex, more men (75%) returned than women (67%). These studies highlight that although there may be a link between sport and return to sport, due to a lack of high-quality research, current literature was unable to come to any conclusion.[47]

Reduced return to sport rates can be attributed to many factors, including age, sex, preinjury activity level, fear, and psychological readiness. Age and sex are 2 variables that have been identified in multiple studies,[43,46] with men and younger athletes being more likely to return to sport. Age may be a proxy measure for changing priorities (ie, family), commitments (ie, employment), and/or opportunities to play at the same level (ie, no longer have the competitive structure of high school, college, or club sports).[43] Furthermore, it has been hypothesized that "For those athletes whose life and social networks are inherently structure around participating in sport, a stronger sense of athletic identity may be a positive motivator for return to sport."[43] Although this hypothesis remains to be tested, this could explain the higher rates of return to sport in younger and elite/professional level athletes. Dunn and Spindler[48] found that higher level of activity before injury and a lower body mass index were predictive of higher activity levels at 2 years following ACLR. Ardern and colleagues[43] found that elite athletes were more likely to return to sport than lower-level athletes.[43] Professional and elite-level athletes may have access to more resources, particularly related to rehabilitation services, but motivation to return to that high level of play and athletic identity may also drive such return to sport. Interestingly, Shah and colleagues[42] found that in NFL players return to play was predicted by draft round. Athletes drafted in the first 4 rounds of the NFL draft were 12.2 times more likely to return to sport than those athletes drafted later or as free agents; this could represent the perceived talent of the player as well as the investment of the organization in that player.[42]

Despite common misconceptions, nonoperatively managed athletes can return to sport without the need for reconstruction.[26] Fitzgerald and colleagues[26] reported a decision-making scheme for returning ACL-deficient athletes to sport in the near term, without furthering of meniscal or articular cartilage injury. There is a paucity of long-term evidence, however, on nonoperatively managed athletes returning to high-level sports. Grindem and colleagues[19] compared return to sport in operatively and nonoperatively managed athletes after ACL injury. They found no significant differences between groups in level I sports participation, and higher level II sports participation in the nonoperative group in the first year after injury. Grindem's study is the only study to the authors' knowledge comparing return to sport rates in the longer term. Further research is needed on long-term nonoperatively managed athletes after ACL injury.

REINJURY

Second injury, whether it is an insult to the ipsilateral graft or the contralateral ACL, is a growing problem after ACLR because rates appear to be higher than once thought. Risk factors for second injury include younger athletes[49] who return to high-level sporting activities early,[50,51] with women having a higher risk of contralateral injury,[52,53] and men having a higher risk of ipsilateral injury.[54,55] Although second injury rates in the general population 5 years after reconstruction are reported to be 6%,[56] rates in young athletes are considerably higher.[51] Paterno and colleagues[51] followed 78 athletes after ACLR and 47 controls over a 24-month period. They found an overall second injury rate of 29.5%, which was an incidence rate nearly 4 times that of the controls (8%). More than 50% of these injuries occurred within the first 72 athletic exposures, whereas in the control group, only 25% were injured within the same time frame.[51] The MOON cohort reported a 20% second injury rate in women and a 5.5% rate in men of 100 soccer players returning to sport after ACLR.[46] Shelbourne and colleagues[55] and Leys and colleagues[57] reported 17% second injury rates in younger athletes. Besides missing more athletic time, increasing health care costs, and increased psychological distress, reinjury and subsequent revision surgery have significantly worse outcomes compared with those after initial reconstruction (**Fig. 2**).[34]

DISCUSSION

ACLR continues to be the gold-standard treatment of ACL injuries in the young athletic population. A survey of American Academy of Orthopedic Surgeons reported 98% of surgeons would recommend surgery if a patient wishes to return to sport, with 79% thinking that ACL-deficient patients are unable to return to all recreational sporting activities without reconstruction.[5] Revisiting the successful outcomes criterion after ACL injury, a successful outcome is considered no reinjury or recurrent giving way, no joint effusion, quadriceps strength symmetry, restored activity level and function, and returning to preinjury sports.[10] After reviewing the current literature and looking at these criteria, counseling athletes to undergo early reconstruction after ACL injury may not be in the athlete's best interest. Undergoing reconstruction does not guarantee athletes return to their preinjury sport, and return to the preinjury competitive level of sport is unlikely. The risk of a second injury is high in young athletes returning to sport, especially in the near term. The risk of secondary injury increases for the contralateral limb in women or the ipsilateral limb in men. The risk for developing osteoarthritis is high in the long term regardless of surgical intervention, and even higher if a revision procedure is required.[58] A *Cochrane Review* found that there was insufficient evidence to recommend ACLR compared with nonoperative treatment, and recent randomized, controlled trials have found no difference between those who had ACLR and those treated nonoperatively with regard to knee function, health status, and return to preinjury activity level and sport after 2 and 5 years in young, active individuals.[19,37,59] With no differences in outcomes between early reconstruction, delayed reconstruction, and no surgery at all, counseling should start by considering nonoperative management. Eitzen and Moksnes[60] found a 5-week progressive exercise program after ACL injury led to significantly improved knee function before deciding to undergo reconstruction or remain nonoperatively managed (**Fig. 3**). The authors reported good compliance with few adverse events during training. Nonoperative management is a viable evidence-based option after ACL injury, allowing some

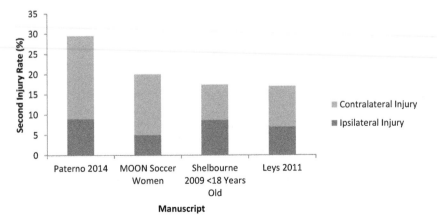

Fig. 2. Second ACL injury rates after ACLR.

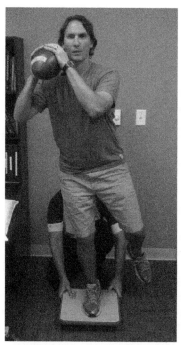

Fig. 3. Unilateral rollerboard portion of perturbation training. The athlete attempts to maintain balance in slight knee flexion while the therapist performs manual perturbations. Progression includes adding sport-specific tasks while maintaining balance.

athletes to return to sport despite being ACL-deficient, with equivalent functional outcomes to those after ACLR. Given there is no evidence in outcomes to undergo early ACLR, nonoperative management should be a first line of treatment choice in athletes after ACL injury (**Table 2**).

Table 2	
Decision-making scheme for ACL deficient athletes	
Test	**Criteria**
Global rating of perceived knee function	$\geq$60%
KOS-ADLS	$\geq$80%
Episodes of giving way	$\leq$1
Timed hop limb symmetry index	$\geq$80%

Global rating of perceived knee function (GRS) is a scale from 0 to 100 asking the athlete to rate their current knee function, with 100 being back to all preinjury activity and function. KOS-ADLS is a patient-reported outcome measure evaluating knee function within daily activity. Episodes of giving way are true moments of instability in which a shifting occurs in the tibiofemoral joint, resulting in an increase in knee pain and joint effusion. The timed hop is one component of hop testing in which the athlete unilaterally hops down a 6-m line as fast as possible. Symmetry index is calculated by dividing the uninvolved limb time by the involved limb time and multiplying by 100.

Data from Fitzgerald GK, Axe MJ, Snyder-Mackler L. A decision-making scheme for returning patients to high-level activity with nonoperative treatment after anterior cruciate ligament rupture. Knee Surg Sports Traumatol Arthrosc 2000;8(2):76–82.

REFERENCES

1. Griffin LY, Albohm MJ, Arendt EA, et al. Understanding and preventing noncontact anterior cruciate ligament injuries: a review of the Hunt Valley II meeting, January 2005. Am J Sports Med 2006;34(9):1512–32. http://dx.doi.org/10.1177/0363546506286866.
2. Hughes G, Watkins J. A risk-factor model for anterior cruciate ligament injury. Sports Med 2006;36(5):411–28. Available at: http://www.ncbi.nlm.nih.gov/pubmed/16646629.
3. Kim S, Bosque J, Meehan JP, et al. Increase in outpatient knee arthroscopy in the United States: a comparison of National Surveys of Ambulatory Surgery, 1996 and 2006. J Bone Joint Surg Am 2011;93(11):994–1000. http://dx.doi.org/10.2106/JBJS.I.01618.
4. Myklebust G, Bahr R. Return to play guidelines after anterior cruciate ligament surgery. Br J Sports Med 2005;39(3):127–31. http://dx.doi.org/10.1136/bjsm.2004.010900.
5. Marx RG, Jones EC, Angel M, et al. Beliefs and attitudes of members of the American Academy of Orthopaedic Surgeons regarding the treatment of anterior cruciate ligament injury. Arthroscopy 2003;19(7):762–70. http://dx.doi.org/10.1016/S0749-8063(03)00398-0.
6. Smith TO, Davies L, Hing CB. Early versus delayed surgery for anterior cruciate ligament reconstruction: a systematic review and meta-analysis. Knee Surg Sports Traumatol Arthrosc 2010;18(3):304–11. http://dx.doi.org/10.1007/s00167-009-0965-z.
7. Shelbourne KD, Foulk DA. Timing of surgery in acute anterior cruciate ligament tears on the return of quadriceps muscle strength after reconstruction using an autogenous patellar tendon graft. Am J Sports Med 1995;23(6):686–9.
8. Andernord D, Karlsson J, Musahl V, et al. Timing of surgery of the anterior cruciate ligament. Arthroscopy 2013;29(11):1863–71. http://dx.doi.org/10.1016/j.arthro.2013.07.270.
9. Gobbi A, Francisco R. Factors affecting return to sports after anterior cruciate ligament reconstruction with patellar tendon and hamstring graft: a prospective clinical investigation. Knee Surg Sports Traumatol Arthrosc 2006;14(10):1021–8. http://dx.doi.org/10.1007/s00167-006-0050-9.
10. Lynch AD, Logerstedt DS, Grindem H, et al. Consensus criteria for defining "successful outcome" after ACL injury and reconstruction: a Delaware-Oslo ACL cohort investigation. Br J Sports Med 2013;1–9. http://dx.doi.org/10.1136/bjsports-2013-092299.
11. De Jong SN, van Caspel DR, van Haeff MJ, et al. Functional assessment and muscle strength before and after reconstruction of chronic anterior cruciate ligament lesions. Arthroscopy 2007;23(1):21–8. http://dx.doi.org/10.1016/j.arthro.2006.08.024, 28.e1–3.
12. Eitzen I, Holm I, Risberg MA. Preoperative quadriceps strength is a significant predictor of knee function two years after anterior cruciate ligament reconstruction. Br J Sports Med 2009;43(5):371–6. http://dx.doi.org/10.1136/bjsm.2008.057059.
13. Palmieri-Smith RM, Thomas AC, Wojtys EM. Maximizing quadriceps strength after ACL reconstruction. Clin Sports Med 2008;27(3):405–24. http://dx.doi.org/10.1016/j.csm.2008.02.001, vii–ix.
14. Logerstedt D, Lynch A, Axe MJ, et al. Symmetry restoration and functional recovery before and after anterior cruciate ligament reconstruction. Knee Surg Sports

Traumatol Arthrosc 2013;21(4):859–68. http://dx.doi.org/10.1007/s00167-012-1929-2.

15. Paterno MV, Ford KR, Myer GD, et al. Limb asymmetries in landing and jumping 2 years following anterior cruciate ligament reconstruction. Clin J Sport Med 2007; 17(4):258–62. http://dx.doi.org/10.1097/JSM.0b013e31804c77ea.

16. Roewer BD, Di Stasi SL, Snyder-Mackler L. Quadriceps strength and weight acceptance strategies continue to improve two years after anterior cruciate ligament reconstruction. J Biomech 2011;44(10):1948–53. http://dx.doi.org/10.1016/j.jbiomech.2011.04.037.

17. Logerstedt D, Lynch A, Axe MJ, et al. Pre-operative quadriceps strength predicts IKDC2000 scores 6 months after anterior cruciate ligament reconstruction. Knee 2013;20(3):208–12. http://dx.doi.org/10.1016/j.knee.2012.07.011.

18. Otzel DM, Chow JW, Tillman MD. Long-term deficits in quadriceps strength and activation following anterior cruciate ligament reconstruction. Phys Ther Sport 2014;1–7. http://dx.doi.org/10.1016/j.ptsp.2014.02.003.

19. Grindem H, Eitzen I, Engebretsen L, et al. Nonsurgical or surgical treatment of ACL injuries: knee function, sports participation, and knee reinjury: the Delaware-Oslo ACL Cohort Study. J Bone Joint Surg Am 2014;96:1233–41. http://dx.doi.org/10.2106/JBJS.M.01054.

20. Ageberg E, Thomeé R, Neeter C, et al. Muscle strength and functional performance in patients with anterior cruciate ligament injury treated with training and surgical reconstruction or training only: a two to five-year followup. Arthritis Rheum 2008;59(12):1773–9. http://dx.doi.org/10.1002/art.24066.

21. Neeter C, Gustavsson A, Thomeé P, et al. Development of a strength test battery for evaluating leg muscle power after anterior cruciate ligament injury and reconstruction. Knee Surg Sports Traumatol Arthrosc 2006;14(6):571–80. http://dx.doi.org/10.1007/s00167-006-0040-y.

22. Tsepis E, Vagenas G, Ristanis S, et al. Thigh muscle weakness in ACL-deficient knees persists without structured rehabilitation. Clin Orthop Relat Res 2006;450: 211–8. http://dx.doi.org/10.1097/01.blo.0000223977.98712.30.

23. Ageberg E, Pettersson A, Fridén T. 15-year follow-up of neuromuscular function in patients with unilateral nonreconstructed anterior cruciate ligament injury initially treated with rehabilitation and activity modification: a longitudinal prospective study. Am J Sports Med 2007;35(12):2109–17. http://dx.doi.org/10.1177/0363546507305018.

24. Muaidi QI, Nicholson LL, Refshauge KM, et al. Prognosis of conservatively managed anterior cruciate ligament injury: a systematic review. Sports Med 2007;37(8):703–16. Available at: http://www.ncbi.nlm.nih.gov/pubmed/17645372.

25. Tagesson S, Oberg B, Good L, et al. A comprehensive rehabilitation program with quadriceps strengthening in closed versus open kinetic chain exercise in patients with anterior cruciate ligament deficiency: a randomized clinical trial evaluating dynamic tibial translation and muscle function. Am J Sports Med 2008; 36(2):298–307. http://dx.doi.org/10.1177/0363546507307867.

26. Fitzgerald GK, Axe MJ, Snyder-Mackler L. A decision-making scheme for returning patients to high-level activity with nonoperative treatment after anterior cruciate ligament rupture. Knee Surg Sports Traumatol Arthrosc 2000;8(2):76–82. http://dx.doi.org/10.1007/s001670050190.

27. Fitzgerald GK, Axe MJ, Snyder-Mackler L. Proposed practice guidelines for nonoperative anterior cruciate ligament rehabilitation of physically active individuals. J Orthop Sports Phys Ther 2000;30(4):194–203. http://dx.doi.org/10.2519/jospt.2000.30.4.194.

28. Moksnes H, Snyder-Mackler L, Risberg MA. Individuals with an anterior cruciate ligament-deficient knee classified as noncopers may be candidates for nonsurgical rehabilitation. J Orthop Sports Phys Ther 2008;38(10):586–95. http://dx.doi.org/10.2519/jospt.2008.2750.
29. Moksnes H, Risberg MA. Performance-based functional evaluation of non-operative and operative treatment after anterior cruciate ligament injury. Scand J Med Sci Sports 2009;19(3):345–55. http://dx.doi.org/10.1111/j.1600-0838.2008.00816.x.
30. Eitzen I, Moksnes H, Snyder-Mackler L, et al. Functional tests should be accentuated more in the decision for ACL reconstruction. Knee Surg Sports Traumatol Arthrosc 2010;18(11):1517–25. http://dx.doi.org/10.1007/s00167-010-1113-5.
31. Keays SL, Bullock-Saxton JE, Keays AC, et al. A 6-year follow-up of the effect of graft site on strength, stability, range of motion, function, and joint degeneration after anterior cruciate ligament reconstruction: patellar tendon versus semitendinosus and Gracilis tendon graft. Am J Sports Med 2007;35(5):729–39. http://dx.doi.org/10.1177/0363546506298277.
32. Hopper DM, Strauss GR, Boyle JJ, et al. Functional recovery after anterior cruciate ligament reconstruction: a longitudinal perspective. Arch Phys Med Rehabil 2008;89(8):1535–41. http://dx.doi.org/10.1016/j.apmr.2007.11.057.
33. Logerstedt DS, Snyder-Mackler L, Ritter RC, et al. Knee stability and movement coordination impairments: knee ligament sprain. J Orthop Sports Phys Ther 2010; 40(4):A1–37. http://dx.doi.org/10.2519/jospt.2010.0303.
34. Wright RW, Gill CS, Chen L, et al. Outcome of revision anterior cruciate ligament reconstruction: a systematic review. J Bone Joint Surg Am 2012;94:531–6. http://dx.doi.org/10.2106/JBJS.K.00733.
35. Mauro CS, Irrgang JJ, Williams BA, et al. Loss of extension following anterior cruciate ligament reconstruction: analysis of incidence and etiology using IKDC criteria. Arthroscopy 2008;24(2):146–53. http://dx.doi.org/10.1016/j.arthro.2007.08.026.
36. Spindler KP, Huston LJ, Wright RW, et al. The prognosis and predictors of sports function and activity at minimum 6 years after anterior cruciate ligament reconstruction a population cohort study. Am J Sports Med 2010;1–12. http://dx.doi.org/10.1177/0363546510383481.
37. Frobell RB, Roos HP, Roos EM, et al. Treatment for acute anterior cruciate ligament tear: five year outcome of randomised trial. BMJ 2013;346:f232. http://dx.doi.org/10.1136/bmj.f232.
38. Logerstedt DS, Snyder-Mackler L, Ritter RC, et al. Knee pain and mobility impairments: meniscal and articular cartilage lesions. J Orthop Sports Phys Ther 2010; 40(6):A1–35. http://dx.doi.org/10.2519/jospt.2010.0304.
39. Barenius B, Ponzer S, Shalabi A, et al. Increased risk of osteoarthritis after anterior cruciate ligament reconstruction: a 14-year follow-up study of a randomized controlled trial. Am J Sports Med 2014;42(5):1049–57. http://dx.doi.org/10.1177/0363546514526139.
40. Chalmers PN, Mall NA, Moric M, et al. Does ACL reconstruction alter natural history?: a systematic literature review of long-term outcomes. J Bone Joint Surg Am 2014;96:292–300. http://dx.doi.org/10.2106/JBJS.L.01713.
41. Bradley JP, Klimkiewicz JJ, Rytel MJ, et al. Anterior cruciate ligament injuries in the National Football League: epidemiology and current treatment trends among team physicians. Arthroscopy 2002;18(5):502–9. http://dx.doi.org/10.1053/jars.2002.30649.
42. Shah VM, Andrews JR, Fleisig GS, et al. Return to play after anterior cruciate ligament reconstruction in National Football League athletes. Am J Sports Med 2010;38(11):2233–9. http://dx.doi.org/10.1177/0363546510372798.

43. Ardern CL, Taylor NF, Feller JA, et al. Fifty-five per cent return to competitive sport following anterior cruciate ligament reconstruction surgery: an updated systematic review and meta-analysis including aspects of physical functioning and contextual factors. Br J Sports Med 2014;48:1543–52. http://dx.doi.org/10.1136/bjsports-2013-093398.

44. McCullough KA, Phelps KD, Spindler KP, et al. Return to high school- and college-level football after anterior cruciate ligament reconstruction: a Multicenter Orthopaedic Outcomes Network (MOON) cohort study. Am J Sports Med 2012; 40(11):2523–9. http://dx.doi.org/10.1177/0363546512456836.

45. Shelbourne KD, Sullivan AN, Bohard K, et al. Return to basketball and soccer after anterior cruciate ligament reconstruction in competitive school-aged athletes. Sports Health 2009;1(3):236–41. http://dx.doi.org/10.1177/1941738109334275.

46. Brophy RH, Schmitz L, Wright RW, et al. Return to play and future ACL injury risk after ACL reconstruction in soccer athletes from the Multicenter Orthopaedic Outcomes Network (MOON) group. Am J Sports Med 2012;40(11):2517–22. http://dx.doi.org/10.1177/0363546512459476.

47. Warner SJ, Smith MV, Wright RW, et al. Sport-specific outcomes after anterior cruciate ligament reconstruction. Arthroscopy 2011;27(8):1129–34. http://dx.doi.org/10.1016/j.arthro.2011.02.022.

48. Dunn WR, Spindler KP. Predictors of activity level 2 years after anterior cruciate ligament reconstruction (ACLR): a Multicenter Orthopaedic Outcomes Network (MOON) ACLR cohort study. Am J Sports Med 2010;38(10):2040–50. http://dx.doi.org/10.1177/0363546510370280.

49. Webster KE, Feller JA, Leigh WB, et al. Younger patients are at increased risk for graft rupture and contralateral injury after anterior cruciate ligament reconstruction. Am J Sports Med 2014;42(3):641–7. http://dx.doi.org/10.1177/0363546513517540.

50. Laboute E, Savalli L, Puig P, et al. Analysis of return to competition and repeat rupture for 298 anterior cruciate ligament reconstructions with patellar or hamstring tendon autograft in sportspeople. Ann Phys Rehabil Med 2010; 53(10):598–614. http://dx.doi.org/10.1016/j.rehab.2010.10.002.

51. Paterno MV, Rauh MJ, Schmitt LC, et al. Incidence of second ACL injuries 2 years after primary ACL reconstruction and return to sport. Am J Sports Med 2014; 42(7):1567–73. http://dx.doi.org/10.1177/0363546514530088.

52. Wright RW, Dunn WR, Amendola A, et al. Risk of tearing the intact anterior cruciate ligament in the contralateral knee and rupturing the anterior cruciate ligament graft during the first 2 years after anterior cruciate ligament reconstruction: a prospective MOON cohort study. Am J Sports Med 2007;35(7):1131–4. http://dx.doi.org/10.1177/0363546507301318.

53. Paterno MV, Schmitt LC, Ford KR, et al. Biomechanical measures during landing and postural stability predict second anterior cruciate ligament injury after anterior cruciate ligament reconstruction and return to sport. Am J Sports Med 2010; 38(10):1968–78. http://dx.doi.org/10.1177/0363546510376053.

54. Bourke HE, Salmon LJ, Waller A, et al. Survival of the anterior cruciate ligament graft and the contralateral ACL at a minimum of 15 years. Am J Sports Med 2012;40(9):1985–92. http://dx.doi.org/10.1177/0363546512454414.

55. Shelbourne KD, Gray T, Haro M. Incidence of subsequent injury to either knee within 5 years after anterior cruciate ligament reconstruction with patellar tendon autograft. Am J Sports Med 2009;37(2):246–51. http://dx.doi.org/10.1177/0363546508325665.

56. Wright RW, Magnussen RA, Dunn WR, et al. Ipsilateral graft and contralateral ACL rupture at five years or more following ACL reconstruction: a systematic

review. J Bone Joint Surg Am 2011;93(12):1159–65. http://dx.doi.org/10.2106/JBJS.J.00898.

57. Leys T, Salmon L, Waller A, et al. Clinical results and risk factors for reinjury 15 years after anterior cruciate ligament reconstruction: a prospective study of hamstring and patellar tendon grafts. Am J Sports Med 2012;40(3):595–605. http://dx.doi.org/10.1177/0363546511430375.

58. Borchers JR, Kaeding CC, Pedroza AD, et al. Intra-articular findings in primary and revision anterior cruciate ligament reconstruction surgery: a comparison of the MOON and MARS study groups. Am J Sports Med 2011;39(9):1889–93. http://dx.doi.org/10.1177/0363546511406871.

59. Smith TO, Postle K, Penny F, et al. Is reconstruction the best management strategy for anterior cruciate ligament rupture? A systematic review and meta-analysis comparing anterior cruciate ligament reconstruction versus non-operative treatment. Knee 2014;21(2):462–70. http://dx.doi.org/10.1016/j.knee.2013.10.009.

60. Eitzen I, Moksnes PH. A progressive 5-week exercise therapy program leads to significant improvement in knee function early after anterior cruciate ligament injury. J Orthop Sports Phys Ther 2010;40(2):705–21. http://dx.doi.org/10.2510/jospt.2010.3345.

Patellofemoral Pain
Epidemiology, Pathophysiology, and Treatment Options

Marcus A. Rothermich, MD[a,*], Neal R. Glaviano, MEd, ATC[b],
Jiacheng Li, BS[b], Joe M. Hart, PhD[b]

KEYWORDS

- Patellofemoral pain • Anterior knee pain • Treatment options

KEY POINTS

- Patellofemoral pain represents a common and debilitating disease process that is often encountered in primary care and orthopedic outpatient clinics.
- The pathophysiology of patellofemoral pain is often multifactorial.
- Because this disease process often affects a younger, more active patient population, activity level has been linked to its cause and progression.
- Supervised physical therapy is the cornerstone of nonoperative management.
- As patellofemoral pain is a heterogenous injury with multiple contributing factors, it remains a challenge for health care providers to diagnose and treat.

Patients with anterior knee pain present a complex and common problem to health care providers. The diagnosis and treatment of these patients often involve a comprehensive evaluation that includes assessing the chronicity of the pain, the specific location of the complaint, and the previous treatment modalities attempted by the patient. This common diagnosis includes a wide variety of different pathologic abnormalities that can be present independently or concomitantly and cause a spectrum of disabilities for the patient. In the evaluation of a patient with anterior knee pain, it is critical for health care providers to appreciate the epidemiology of the problem, the differential diagnosis of multiple possible pathologic abnormalities generating anterior knee pain, and the various options regarding both operative and nonoperative treatment.

[a] Department of Orthopaedic Surgery, Washington University, Campus Box 8233, St Louis, MO 63108, USA; [b] Department of Orthopaedic Surgery, University of Virginia, 400 Ray C. Hunt Drive, Suite 330, Charlottesville, VA 22903, USA
* Corresponding author.
E-mail address: rothermichm@wudosis.wustl.edu

Clin Sports Med 34 (2015) 313–327
http://dx.doi.org/10.1016/j.csm.2014.12.011
0278-5919/15/$ – see front matter © 2015 Elsevier Inc. All rights reserved.
sportsmed.theclinics.com

EPIDEMIOLOGY
Incidence and Prevalence

Anterior knee pain represents one of the most common diagnoses in pediatric and adult primary care and in orthopedic outpatient clinics.[1–3] Although the prevalence of patellofemoral pain as the primary cause of knee injury has been estimated to be as high as 40%, the annual incidence and true prevalence of patellofemoral pain are unknown.[4] Patients with anterior knee pain range from active pediatric patients to sedentary elderly patients, but a peak of prevalence in patellofemoral pain has been observed in young, active adolescents between the ages of 12 and 17.[4,5] This population most commonly presents in the outpatient clinic with complaints of chronic anterior knee pain with sporting activity.[6] Additional cohorts with a high prevalence of patellofemoral pain include active adults—the so-called weekend warrior—and young military recruits.[5] These populations represent the majority of the patients presenting with patellofemoral pain, but a high prevalence is also noted in the general population.

Gender Differences

In addition to the differences in age and activity level of patients often diagnosed with patellofemoral pain, an important variable in understanding the epidemiology of anterior knee pain is differences in the prevalence between male and female patients. Several epidemiologic studies have demonstrated a higher incidence of patellofemoral pain in female patients.[7–12] This reported female predominance varies, but has been estimated to be as high as a 2-fold higher annual incidence in women compared with men.[4,9] Although the true incidence of patellofemoral pain in the general population is unknown, a recent epidemiologic study in military recruits demonstrated an annual incidence of patellofemoral pain was 33 of 1000 person-years in female patients compared with 15 of 1000 person-years in male patients, demonstrating that female patients were 2.23 times more likely to develop patellofemoral pain annually during the study period.[9] The established prevalence of patellofemoral pain in this population showed a less dramatic difference, with a reported prevalence of 15.3% in female patients and 12.3% in male patients in their cohort of military recruits.[9] Studies have also shown a similar prevalence in athletes, with long-term follow-up typically demonstrating a longer and more refractory course in female patients.[1]

Quality of Life

An important element in the treatment of patients with patellofemoral pain is an understanding of the impact that chronic anterior knee pain can have on the quality of life that a patient experiences.[13–15] A 2013 study by Cheung and colleagues[13] evaluated the relative relationship between patellofemoral pain and subjective quality of life in both recreational and professional athletes. This study assessed several elements of the Medical Outcomes Study 36-Item Short Form Health Survey (SF-36), including subscales of physical functioning, role limitations due to knee pain, bodily pain, general health perceptions, vitality, social functioning, role limitations due to emotional disturbances, and mental health.[13] They demonstrated a decreased quality of life in each subscale of the SF-36 for patients with patellofemoral pain, most dramatically in bodily pain and vitality for recreational athletes and role limitations due to knee pain for professional athletes.[13] This information is valuable to the physician or other health care provider treating patients with patellofemoral pain. The morbidity of patellofemoral pain includes both physical and mental limitations due to the chronic knee pain. This physical and mental morbidity for patients with patellofemoral pain leads to increased health care costs both directly from nonoperative and operative treatment modalities and indirectly from decreased productivity from these patients.[16]

PATHOPHYSIOLOGY

The patient with anterior knee pain presents a challenge to the treating health care provider in both the diagnosis and the treatment of the pain. An important element in the diagnosis of patellofemoral pain is the exclusion of other possible causes, including intra-articular pathologic abnormality, plica syndromes, Osgood-Schlatter disease, neuromas, and other rare causes.[17] Patellofemoral pain is a diagnosis that describes anterior knee pain that is often multifactorial and caused by a variable combination of malalignment of the lower extremity, muscular imbalance around the hip and knee joints, and overactivity.[17] Each of these causative factors plays an important role in the development of patellofemoral pain.

Malalignment

Malalignment of the lower extremity is a common cause of patellofemoral pain.[17–20] This structural cause of anterior knee pain is often multifactorial and includes an increased Q-angle in the weight-bearing position, genu valgum, tibia varum, and patellar malalignment.[17,20] Patellar stability includes a complex interplay between the alignment of the femur and tibia, the osseous patellofemoral joint geometry, and the soft tissue constraints surrounding the patella.[18] The trochlear groove plays a critical role in osseous patellar stability, and hypoplasia of the trochlea is a common cause of congenital patellar instability.[17–20] This hypoplasia often results in a cascade of pathologic abnormalities that includes patellar malalignment, which leads to instability and dislocation events, often causing chondromalacia patellae.[19] Patellar malalignment and instability are often characterized radiographically by a lateral tilting of the patella on a 45° weight-bearing view of the patellofemoral joint, which is often coexistent with or a precursor to patellofemoral osteoarthritis.[17] These factors of patellofemoral malalignment all play important roles in the pathophysiology of patellofemoral pain.

Muscular Imbalance

Muscular imbalance has been described as an important contributor to the observed patellar maltracking that causes patellofemoral pain.[21] This imbalance includes a loss of muscle volume and strength in the quadriceps, specifically in the vastus medialis obliquus (VMO) muscle.[21] Kaya and colleagues[21] described the asymmetry in VMO volume and strength compared with the asymptomatic limb as well as a delayed onset in the activity of the VMO compared with the vastus lateralis. In addition to the volume and strength of the quadriceps, several studies have described trunk biomechanics as another critical factor in patellofemoral tracking.[22–26] Boling and colleagues[22] demonstrated that patients with patellofemoral pain displayed more weakness in eccentric hip abduction and hip external rotation, allowing for increased hip adduction and internal rotation during functional movements. The relative weakness of the gluteus medius and gluteus maximus in patients with patellofemoral pain increases ipsilateral lean, subjecting the patient to large external forces in the sagittal and transverse planes.[23] This dynamic imbalance places increased demand on the quadriceps and has been postulated to cause increased patellofemoral joint compression, exacerbating the dynamic patellar maltracking and accelerating patellofemoral joint osteoarthritic changes.[23]

Overactivity

Overactivity is often a contributing factor to the development of patellofemoral pain.[27] As the epidemiologic studies reviewed demonstrate, the highest prevalence of patellofemoral pain occurs in young, active patients.[4,5] Also, a rapid acceleration of activity through athletic conditioning or military training often results in the development of patellofemoral pain in adults. A classic study by Milgrom and colleagues[27] evaluated a large cohort of infantry recruits and reported a high incidence of patellofemoral pain that increased throughout a standard military training course. The common contributors to patellofemoral pain in most individuals—malalignment, muscle imbalance, and overactivity—play important roles in the complex pathophysiology in patients with anterior knee pain.

RISK FACTORS

A multitude of anthropometric, anatomic, neuromuscular, and lower extremity movement patterns has been examined to identify those at the greatest risk for developing patellofemoral pain.[20,28,29] Prospective studies have identified risk factors being predominantly intrinsic in nature and the modification of these impairments are often the focus during the rehabilitation process to minimize the development of this debilitating condition.[4,30]

Anthropometric measurements have been postulated to increase the potential risk for individuals developing patellofemoral pain. Several variables, such as height, mass, body mass index, body fat percentage, age, and somatotype, have been examined but have not been found to be a significant risk factor.[4,9,29–32]

Anatomic factors have been found to have strong correlations to an increased risk of developing patellofemoral pain, such as soft tissue restrictions and lower extremity alignment.[28,30] Soft tissue restriction, such as tightness of the quadriceps, hamstrings, triceps surae, and iliotibial band, have all been found within a population with patellofemoral pain and have been theorized to alter arthrokinematics, which may increase patellofemoral joint stress.[4,28,33–37] Although these restrictions have been suggested for targeted rehabilitation interventions, isolated muscle flexibility programs have not been studied to date.[38] Lower extremity alignment due to increased navicular drop and tibial torsion has also been seen to have an influence on increasing lateral patellofemoral joint stress.[30,39,40] The utilization of orthotics has been found to improve lower extremity alignment and has also been shown to both improve functional performance and decrease pain in patients who suffer from patellofemoral pain.[41–43]

Altered neuromuscular function of the lower extremity has been identified in patients with patellofemoral pain, with common muscle weakness in the knee extensors, knee flexors, and hip abductors.[4,20,30–32,44–46] Isokinetic knee extensor weakness significantly predicted the development of future cases of patellofemoral pain.[32,47,48] Also, individuals suffering from patellofemoral pain often experience gluteus medius weakness in both hip abduction and external rotation compared with healthy controls.[22,49,50] This weakness has been theorized to correlate to increased hip adduction during functional tasks, which may increase the patellofemoral joint stress in these individuals.[24,40,51] However, a recent systematic review examining prospective studies[45] questioned the association between hip muscle strength and the development of patellofemoral pain, suggesting that gluteus medius weakness may be a sequela of the pathologic abnormality rather than a predisposition; this is an area of controversy that warrants further research. Although gluteus medius strength may not be solely related to the increased hip adduction, electromyographic evidence suggests individuals with patellofemoral pain present with altered muscle activation.[52,53]

A delay in the onset of activation and a decrease in the duration of gluteus medius activation during functional tasks have been suggested to play a role in frontal plane motion; this is an area for future research.[49,52–54]

Prospective trials have also found additional factors that increase the risk of developing patellofemoral pain during functional activities, such as a jump-landing task. Landing biomechanics were examined in 13-year-old and 16-year-old female adolescents, and an increased risk of developing patellofemoral pain was found when knee abduction moments were greater than 15 Nm and 25 Nm, respectfully.[55,56] Increased risk of patellofemoral pain development was also found with a decrease in peak knee flexion angle during landing and a decreased vertical ground reaction force.[4] These altered functional tasks support using movement pattern modifications during rehabilitation to improve landing biomechanics, decrease pain, and improve functional limitations.[57–59]

OPERATIVE MANAGEMENT

For most patients with patellofemoral pain, surgical intervention is not indicated. Surgery is typically only considered when patients have been refractory to nonoperative management for 6 to 12 months.[60] Interventions must be justified by precise indications, including a clearly defined abnormality that the operation can specifically target (eg, identifiable lesion or patellofemoral imbalance).[61,62] The 3 general surgical options include patellar realignment, resurfacing, and arthroplasty.

Realignment

Lateral release is a proximal realignment procedure most appropriate for patients presenting with a tight lateral retinaculum and lateral patellar tilt.[60,61] This procedure is minimally invasive, using arthroscopy or combined with a mini-open approach.[61] Pain and instability due to medial patellar subluxation is a serious complication, often arising after an aggressive release.[61,62] Some patients may require additional realignment procedures, including proximal imbrication or reconstruction of the medial patellofemoral ligament.[61] Early motion of the knee is essential to avoid postoperative stiffness.[61]

Tibial osteotomies are used as distal realignment procedures and are most appropriate for patients with lateral malalignment accompanied by lateral and distal patellar facet lesions.[60,61] Patients with patellofemoral pain are often successfully treated with a medial tibial tubercle transfer.[61] Anteromedial transfer is another surgical option that decreases overall patellar load and reduces postoperative stiffness.[61] Full weight-bearing should be avoided for 6 weeks to allow for healing of the osteotomy.[61,62] Distal realignment procedures are generally contraindicated for proximal and medial patellar facet lesions.[61]

Resurfacing

Cartilage restoration procedures, including autologous chondrocyte implantation (ACI-C) and osteochondral transfers, have seen mixed success in the population of patients with patellofemoral pain caused by a defect in the cartilage of the patellofemoral joint.[62] A 2012 study by Macmull and colleagues[63] of 48 patients with chondromalacia patellae receiving autologous chondrocyte implantation (ACI-C) for large patellar defects showed good to excellent outcomes for roughly half the subjects with either autologous chondrocyte implantation (ACI-C) or matrix-carried autologous chondrocyte implantation (MACI) procedures. Less invasive options, including chondroplasty, microfracture, and abrasion, may offer equivalent benefit and should be used preferentially, with the possible exception of patients with large cartilage defects.[62]

Other Surgical Interventions

A final, aggressive surgical option includes patellofemoral arthroplasty, which may be indicated in cases of end-stage osteoarthritic degeneration, and can enable a return to sporting activity with some limitations.[61,64]

The effectiveness of surgical interventions for patellofemoral pain remains difficult to assess, because most available studies are uncontrolled case series. A 2007 randomized controlled study by Kettunen and colleagues[65] of 56 patients with chronic patellofemoral pain found that treatment with arthroscopy in addition to an 8-week home exercise program did not result in a better outcome than treatment with exercise alone. Patients were matched for baseline characteristics including symptom duration and work-related physical loading.[65] The conclusion remained the same in a 5-year follow-up,[66] although it is notable that improvements persisted for most subjects who had improved in the initial study.

Another emerging surgical option is patellofemoral trochleoplasty to treat patients with patellofemoral dysplasia by deepening the trochlear groove.[67–70] This procedure has shown good short-term outcomes for patients with dysplasia; however, little high-level evidence is available to support long term efficacy.

NONOPERATIVE MANAGEMENT

Although many patients with patellofemoral pain may improve with surgical management, nonoperative treatment remains the mainstay for the initial management of this common problem. The spectrum of nonoperative management options includes a wide variety of various treatment modalities. Patellar taping, bracing, pharmacologics, and the use of therapeutic ultrasound are nonoperative treatment options that are controversial in the literature and have not been universally accepted.[71] Physical therapy, however, has been shown in several systematic reviews and meta-analyses to result satisfactorily in a majority of patients with patellofemoral pain.[72–77] The use of physical therapy in the treatment of patellofemoral pain is the most widely accepted initial route of management. A recent systematic review by Frye and colleagues[74] demonstrated that exercise interventions for patients with patellofemoral pain are effective in the immediate decrease in pain and increase in function. There is no consensus, however, on the most effective physical therapy modalities or specific treatment protocols. This controversy has existed for decades, and recent research has added to the vast literature on the subject of the nonoperative management of patellofemoral pain.

Because the cause of patellofemoral pain has been described as a multifactorial process that includes altered lower extremity biomechanics, local joint impairments, and overactivity, the nonoperative management of this difficult disease process often includes a multimodal treatment strategy.[73] Modalities of management are numerous and most commonly include physical therapy as the cornerstone of the treatment algorithm with the variable supplementation of other methods, including patellar taping, bracing, and neuromuscular electrical stimulation. In patients managed with physical therapy as the primary treatment method, the type of therapy prescribed is also variable and controversial. Different therapy options include open or closed chain exercises, strength training of the hip or knee joints, and flexibility training. This multitude of therapy options comprises the most controversial aspects of the nonoperative treatment of patients with patellofemoral pain.

In reviewing the most controversial topics in current rehabilitation protocols for patients with patellofemoral pain, it is critical to first understand the accepted components of treatment and also the most common modalities used for these patients.

Recent literature has demonstrated an improvement in patients more often when supervised therapy is used rather than home-based therapy programs.[78] Also, patients are most effectively treated when patellofemoral pain is diagnosed and therapy is started early in the disease process.[79] A late or delayed diagnosis of anterior knee pain often delays treatment and leads to a more chronic and debilitating course of patellofemoral pain. A final commonly accepted component of treatment of patients with patellofemoral pain includes the weight-bearing status during therapy. Several studies[80–83] demonstrate improved outcomes in these patients when therapy focuses on a weight-bearing protocol that includes activation of the quadriceps to improve the muscular imbalance that contributes to the pathologic abnormality. Although the type of weight-bearing physical therapy is controversial, the weight-bearing nature of the activity itself is widely accepted as critical to the success of the protocol.

Patellar Taping and Bracing

In addition to physical therapy, several other treatment modalities are commonly used either in isolation or as a supplement to the therapy protocol. The use of patellar taping and bracing is a controversial element in the armamentarium of nonoperative treatment options. Several studies[84–86] have demonstrated the efficacy of patellar taping and bracing in the reduction of pain and the improvement of postural and functional control. Aminaka and Gribble[84] demonstrated reduced pain and improved performance in patients with patellar taping who underwent a star excursion balance test, a measure of dynamic postural control.[87] The taping of the patellofemoral joint is designed to provide a mechanical shift to the patella and improve tracking within the trochlear groove.[85] Traditional nonelastic tape and more modern elastic Kinesio Tape have been used in this treatment modality, often with a successful reduction of pain and improvement of dynamic postural control.[85] However, studies[85,86] have demonstrated that the pain reduction and functional improvement are often not significant enough to be clinically relevant for most patients. The timing of the tape application and its beneficial effects remains controversial.[86]

Neuromuscular Electrical Stimulation

Another debated modality in the treatment of patellofemoral pain is the use of neuromuscular electrical stimulation.[88,89] This method of treatment includes electrically induced muscle contraction that can be used to supplement or replace voluntary contraction during physical therapy.[88] Proponents of the use of neuromuscular electrical stimulation argue that its use can be part of a home-based therapy regimen that is more cost-effective and often more convenient for patients.[88] Also, studies[88,89] have demonstrated an improvement in the force-generating capacity of the VMO in patients who have undergone neuromuscular electrical stimulation. However, its use in isolation has not been shown to surpass the efficacy of a formal, supervised physical therapy program. It is not widely accepted as a replacement for physical therapy and remains a controversial complement to physical therapy in the treatment of patients with patellofemoral pain.

Open Versus Closed Chain Exercises

Although patellar taping, bracing, and neuromuscular electrical stimulation are debated elements of nonoperative management, the use of physical therapy is universally accepted as the benchmark of treatment for patients with patellofemoral pain. Physical therapy often incorporates open or closed chain exercises.[48,90] Open chain exercises, which are non-weight-bearing such as resisted leg extensions, have long been used in strengthening the quadriceps muscle. However, these exercises have been shown to exacerbate the symptoms in patients with patellofemoral pain.[48] Closed chain exercises are weight-bearing and hence re-create the functional position of many daily activities that are used in physical therapy protocols.[48] Witvrouw and colleagues[48] conducted a prospective, randomized study that evaluated the efficacy of open versus closed kinetic chain exercises in the nonoperative management of patients with patellofemoral pain. This study included 60 patients who were randomized to a 5-week physical therapy program consisting of either open or closed chain exercises and demonstrated significant functional improvements in both groups of patients.[48] These similar significant improvements were also seen in a 5-year follow-up of the same cohort of patients.[90] This study supports using closed chain exercises, but also demonstrates significant improvement in patients using open chain exercises. Although closed chain therapy protocols remain more popular and more widely used because of similarities with functional activities, considerable controversy remains regarding the most optimal physical therapy modality.

Strengthening

Strengthening is an important element of a physical therapy program and often focuses on the improved activation and strength of the quadriceps muscles. However, strengthening of the hip and abdominal musculature is also critical in the treatment of patellofemoral pain. A recent systematic review by Peters and Tyson[91] demonstrated moderate-quality to high-quality evidence that therapy protocols that target the abdominal and hip muscular groups provide relief of pain and improved function. An additional case series by Earl and Hoch[92] and a randomized controlled trial by Nakagawa and colleagues[93] report similar improvements in functional outcomes with the addition of hip abductor and abdominal strengthening to standardized quadriceps-strengthening therapy protocols. The randomized controlled trial assigned patients to either an isolated quadriceps-strengthening program or a program that included hip abductor and abdominal strengthening and demonstrated a significant improvement in pain in patients with the additional hip and abdominal strengthening.[93] Resisted strengthening of the hip abductors and external rotators has also been shown to alter lower extremity joint loading and improve lower extremity biomechanics while running.[94,95] Also, gluteal muscle strengthening improves pelvis stability and both static and dynamic postural control.[96,97] Although many studies demonstrate pain reduction and improved functional status in patients with patellofemoral pain with the addition of hip and abdominal muscle strengthening, there is inconclusive evidence regarding the efficacy of individual strengthening exercises and the ideal strengthening regimen remains controversial.[96]

In addition to hip and core strengthening, physical therapy protocols that focus on strengthening of the quadriceps muscles remain a critical element in nonoperative treatment. A systematic review by Kooiker and colleagues[98] emphasized the importance of quadriceps strengthening. This study demonstrated evidence for the effectiveness of isolated quadriceps strengthening in pain reduction and functional improvement and recommended that strengthening of the quadriceps be included in physical therapy protocols to address patellofemoral pain.[98] Although the literature supports physical therapy protocols including quadriceps strengthening, there is no consensus regarding the specific mode or frequency of these exercises.

Flexibility

A final important element of physical therapy for the treatment of patellofemoral pain includes the flexibility of the soft tissues. Tissue tightness, specifically in the anterior hip musculature, quadriceps, hamstrings, iliotibial band, and gastrocnemius, can influence and contribute to patellofemoral pain. A case-control study[28] demonstrated poorer flexibility of the gastrocnemius, soleus, quadriceps, and hamstrings in patients with patellofemoral pain compared with control subjects. The results of this study suggest that flexibility training be included as a supplement to strengthening in physical therapy protocols.

A recent systematic review[7] outlined important elements of the effects of physical therapy on decreasing pain and increasing function in patients with patellofemoral pain. Although patients demonstrated decreased Visual Analog Scale pain scores and increased Kujala functional outcome scores at the conclusion of the physical therapy program, these improved patient outcomes diminished over time, suggesting that the benefits of physical therapy were lost once the patients stopped exercising. These results are important in guiding health care providers managing patients with a nonoperative treatment regimen. The temporary nature of the beneficial effects of therapy suggests that a comprehensive strengthening approach should be considered to include strengthening of the quadriceps, hip, and abdominal musculature as well as supplemental flexibility training. Also, these patients should be counseled to continue regular exercises at home after the formal physical therapy program is complete.

SUMMARY

Patellofemoral pain represents a common and debilitating disease process that is often encountered in primary care and orthopedic outpatient clinics. The pathophysiology of patellofemoral pain is often multifactorial. Malalignment of the lower extremity and an increased Q-angle often contribute to the cause of anterior knee pain. Also, a muscular imbalance can lead to decreased stability of the patellofemoral joint with normal weight-bearing activities. A decrease in the strength of the VMO most commonly causes an asymmetry of biomechanical forces acting on the knee, and this muscular imbalance has been implicated in the pathophysiology of patellofemoral pain. Finally, overactivity has been demonstrated as a factor in the development of patellofemoral pain. As this disease process often affects a younger, more active patient population, activity level has been linked to its cause and progression.

Although several operative procedures have been successfully used in patients with patellofemoral pain, nonoperative management remains the most commonly used initial treatment course. Supervised physical therapy is the cornerstone of nonoperative management. Most of the current literature supports the use of closed chain, weight-bearing exercises for a successful physical therapy program. However, the use of patellar taping, bracing, and neuromuscular electrical stimulation remains controversial. Also, strengthening of the hip and abdominal musculature and flexibility training are generally favored but may not be universally accepted. Considerable debate continues on the specific exercises, target muscles, and duration of an ideal physical therapy regimen for patients with patellofemoral pain. As patellofemoral pain is a heterogenous injury with multiple contributing factors, it remains a challenge for health care providers to diagnose and treat.

REFERENCES

1. Blond L, Hansen L. Patellofemoral pain syndrome in athletes: a 5.7-year retrospective follow-up study of 250 athletes. Acta Orthop Belg 1998;64(4): 393–400.
2. Witman PA, Melvin M, Nicholas JA. Common problems seen in a metropolitan sports injury clinic. The Physician and Sportsmedicine 1981;9(3):105–8.

3. Wood L, Muller S, Peat G. The epidemiology of patellofemoral disorders in adulthood: a review of routine general practice morbidity. Prim Health Care Res Dev 2011;12(2):157–64.
4. Witvrouw E, Callaghan MJ, Stefanik JJ, et al. Patellofemoral pain: consensus statement from the 3rd International Patellofemoral Pain Research Retreat held in Vancouver, 2013. Br J Sports Med 2014;48:411–4.
5. Callaghan MJ, Selfe J. Has the incidence or prevalence of patellofemoral pain in the general population in the United Kingdom been properly evaluated? Phys Ther Sport 2007;8(1):37–43.
6. Luhmann SJ, Schoenecker PL, Dobbs MB, et al. Adolescent patellofemoral pain: implicating the medial patellofemoral ligament as the main pain generator. J Child Orthop 2008;2:269–77.
7. Barber Foss KD, Myer GD, Chen SS, et al. Expected prevalence from the differential diagnosis of anterior knee pain in adolescent female athletes during pre-participation screening. J Athl Train 2012;47(5):519–24.
8. Barber Foss KD, Myer GD, Magnussen RA, et al. Diagnostic differences for anterior knee pain between sexes in adolescent basketball players. J Athl Enhanc 2014; 3(1):1814.
9. Boling M, Padua D, Marshall S, et al. Gender differences in the incidence and prevalence of patellofemoral pain syndrome. Scand J Med Sci Sports 2010;20: 723–30.
10. Cowan SM, Crossley KM. Does gender influence neuromotor control of the knee and hip? J Electromyogr Kinesiol 2009;19(2):276–82.
11. Myer GD, Ford KR, Barber Foss KD, et al. The incidence and potential pathomechanics of patellofemoral pain in female athletes. Clin Biomech (Bristol, Avon) 2010;25(7):700–7.
12. Nejati P, Forogh B, Moeineddin R, et al. Patellofemoral pain syndrome in Iranian female athletes. Acta Med Iran 2011;49(3):169–72.
13. Cheung RT, Zhang Z, Ngai SP. Different relationships between the level of patellofemoral pain and quality of life in professional and amateur athletes. PM R 2013; 5(7):568–72.
14. Crossley KM, Bennell KL, Cowan SM, et al. Analysis of outcome measures for persons with patellofemoral pain: which are reliable and valid? Arch Phys Med Rehabil 2004;85:815–22.
15. Thomas MJ, Wood L, Selfe J, et al. Anterior knee pain in younger adults as a precursor to subsequent patellofemoral osteoarthritis: a systematic review. BMC Musculoskelet Disord 2010;9(11):201.
16. Swan Tan S, van Linschoten R, van Middelkoop M, et al. Cost-utility of exercise therapy in adolescents and young adults suffering from the patellofemoral pain syndrome. Scand J Med Sci Sports 2010;20(4):568–79.
17. Thomee R, Augustsson J, Karlsson J. Patellofemoral pain syndrome: a review of current issues. Sports Med 1999;28(4):245–62.
18. Chiang Colvin A, West RV. Patellar instability. J Bone Joint Surg Am 2008;90:2751–62.
19. Tuna BK, Semiz-Oysu A, Pekar B, et al. The association of patellofemoral joint morphology with chondromalacia patella: a quantitative MRI analysis. Clin Imaging 2014;38(4):495–8.
20. Lankhorst NE, Bierma-Zeinstra S, van Middelkoop M. Factors associated with patellofemoral pain syndrome: a systematic review. Br J Sports Med 2013;47:193–206.
21. Kaya D, Citaker S, Kerimoglu U, et al. Women with patellofemoral pain syndrome have quadriceps femoris volume and strength deficiency. Knee Surg Sports Traumatol Arthrosc 2011;19:242–7.

22. Boling MC, Padua DA, Creighton RA. Concentric and eccentric torque of the hip musculature in individuals with and without patellofemoral pain. J Athl Train 2009; 44(1):7–13.

23. Nakagawa TH, Maciel CD, Serrao FV. Trunk biomechanics and its association with hip and knee kinematics in patients with and without patellofemoral pain. Man Ther 2015 Feb;20(1):189–93.

24. Nakagawa TH, Moriya ET, Maciel CD, et al. Trunk, pelvis, hip, and knee kinematics, hip strength, and gluteal muscle activation during a single-leg squat in males and females with and without patellofemoral pain syndrome. J Orthop Sports Phys Ther 2012;42(6):491–501.

25. Nakagawa TH, Serrao FV, Maciel CD, et al. Hip and knee kinematics are associated with pain and self-reported functional status in males and females with patellofemoral pain. Int J Sports Med 2013;34(11):997–1002.

26. Rojhani Shirazi Z, Biabani Moghaddam M, Motealleh A. Comparative evaluation of core muscle recruitment pattern in response to sudden external perturbations in patients with patellofemoral pain syndrome and healthy subjects. Arch Phys Med Rehabil 2014;95(7):1383–9.

27. Milgrom C, Finestone A, Eldad A, et al. Patellofemoral pain caused by overactivity. J Bone Joint Surg Am 1991;73A(7):1041–3.

28. Piva SR, Goodnite EA, Childs JD. Strength around the hip and flexibility of soft tissues in individuals with and without patellofemoral pain syndrome. J Orthop Sports Phys Ther 2005;35(12):793–801.

29. Waryasz GR, McDermott AY. Patellofemoral pain syndrome (PFPS): a systematic review of anatomy and potential risk factors. Dyn Med 2008;7:9. http://dx.doi.org/ 10.1186/1476-5918-7-9.

30. Boling MC, Padua DA, Marshall SW, et al. A prospective investigation of biomechanical risk factors for patellofemoral pain syndrome: the joint undertaking to monitor and prevent ACL injury (JUMP-ACL) cohort. Am J Sports Med 2009; 37(11):2108–16.

31. Van Tiggelen D, Cowan S, Coorevits P, et al. Delayed vastus medialis obliquus to vastus lateralis onset timing contributes to the development of patellofemoral pain in previously healthy men: a prospective study. Am J Sports Med 2009;37(6):1099–105.

32. Van Tiggelen D, Witvrouw E, Coorevits P, et al. Analysis of isokinetic parameters in the development of anterior knee pain syndrome: a prospective study in a military setting. Isokinetics Exerc Sci 2004;12:223–8.

33. Halabchi F, Mazaheri R, Seif-Barghi T. Patellofemoral pain syndrome and modifiable intrinsic risk factors; how to assess and address? Asian J Sports Med 2013; 4(2):85–100.

34. White LC, Dolphin P, Dixon J. Hamstring length in patellofemoral pain syndrome. Physiotherapy 2009;95(1):24–8.

35. Whyte EF, Moran K, Shortt CP, et al. The influence of reduced hamstring length on patellofemoral joint stress during squatting in healthy male adults. Gait Posture 2010;31(1):47–51.

36. Rowlands BW, Brantingham JW. The efficacy of patella mobilization in patients suffering from patellofemoral pain syndrome. J Neuromusculoskelet Syst 1999; 7(4):142–9.

37. Hudson Z, Darthuy E. Iliotibial band tightness and patellofemoral pain syndrome: a case-control study. Man Ther 2009;14(2):147–51.

38. Selfe J, Callaghan M, Witvrouw E, et al. Targeted interventions for patellofemoral pain syndrome (TIPPS): classification of clinical subgroups. BMJ Open 2013; 3(9):e003795. http://dx.doi.org/10.1136/bmjopen-2013-003795.

39. Barton CJ, Bonanno D, Levinger P, et al. Foot and ankle characteristics in patellofemoral pain syndrome: a case control and reliability study. J Orthop Sports Phys Ther 2010;40(5):286–96.

40. Noehren B, Pohl MB, Sanchez Z, et al. Proximal and distal kinematics in female runners with patellofemoral pain. Clin Biomech 2012;27(4):366–71.

41. Barton CJ, Menz HB, Crossley KM. The immediate effects of foot orthoses on functional performance in individuals with patellofemoral pain syndrome. Br J Sports Med 2011;45(3):193–7.

42. Collins N, Crossley K, Beller E, et al. Foot orthoses and physiotherapy in the treatment of patellofemoral pain syndrome: randomised clinical trial. Br J Sports Med 2009;43(3):169–71.

43. Sutlive TG, Mitchell SD, Maxfield SN, et al. Identification of individuals with patellofemoral pain whose symptoms improved after a combined program of foot orthosis use and modified activity: a preliminary investigation. Phys Ther 2004;84(1):49–61.

44. Hart JM, Pietrosimone B, Hertel J, et al. Quadriceps activation following knee injuries: a systematic review. J Athl Train 2010;45(1):87–97.

45. Rathleff MS, Rathleff CR, Crossley KM, et al. Is hip strength a risk factor for patellofemoral pain? A systematic review and meta-analysis. Br J Sports Med 2014;48(14):1088. http://dx.doi.org/10.1136/bjsports-2013-093305.

46. Rathleff CR, Baird WN, Olesen JL, et al. Hip and knee strength is not affected in 12-16 year old adolescents with patellofemoral pain–a cross-sectional population-based study. PLoS One 2013;8(11):e79153.

47. Duvigneaud N, Bernard E, Stevens V, et al. Isokinetic assessment of patellofemoral pain syndrome: a prospective study in female recruits. Isokinetics Exerc Sci 2008;16:213–9.

48. Witvrouw E, Lysens R, Bellemans J, et al. Open versus closed kinetic chain exercises for patellofemoral pain. A prospective, randomized study. Am J Sports Med 2000;28(5):687–94.

49. Barton CJ, Lack S, Malliaras P, et al. Gluteal muscle activity and patellofemoral pain syndrome: a systematic review. Br J Sports Med 2013;47(4):207–14.

50. Willson JD, Kernozek TW, Arndt RL, et al. Gluteal muscle activation during running in females with and without patellofemoral pain syndrome. Clin Biomech 2011;26(7):735–40.

51. Noehren B, Hamill J, Davis I. Prospective evidence for a hip etiology in patellofemoral pain. Med Sci Sports Exerc 2013;45(6):1120–4.

52. Nakagawa TH, Muniz TB, Baldon RM, et al. Electromyographic preactivation pattern of the gluteus medius during weight-bearing functional tasks in women with and without anterior knee pain. Rev Bras Fisioter 2011;15(1):59–65.

53. Ott B, Cosby NL, Grindstaff TL, et al. Hip and knee muscle function following aerobic exercise in individuals with patellofemoral pain syndrome. J Electromyogr Kinesiol 2011;21(4):631–7.

54. Souza RB, Powers CM. Differences in hip kinematics, muscle strength, and muscle activation between subjects with and without patellofemoral pain. J Orthop Sports Phys Ther 2009;39(1):12–9.

55. Myer GD, Ford KR, Di Stasi SL, et al. High knee abduction moments are common risk factors for patellofemoral pain (PFP) and anterior cruciate ligament (ACL) injury in girls: is PFP itself a predictor for subsequent ACL injury? Br J Sports Med 2015 Jan;49(2):118–22.

56. Myer GD, Ford KR, Foss KD, et al. A predictive model to estimate knee-abduction moment: implications for development of a clinically applicable patellofemoral pain screening tool in female athletes. J Athl Train 2014;49(3):389–98.

57. Noehren B, Scholz J, Davis I. The effect of real-time gait retraining on hip kinematics, pain and function in subjects with patellofemoral pain syndrome. Br J Sports Med 2011;45(9):691–6.

58. Cheung RT, Davis IS. Landing pattern modification to improve patellofemoral pain in runners: a case series. J Orthop Sports Phys Ther 2011;41(12): 914–9.

59. Willy RW, Davis IS. Varied response to mirror gait retraining of gluteus medius control, hip kinematics, pain, and function in 2 female runners with patellofemoral pain. J Orthop Sports Phys Ther 2013;43(12):864–74.

60. Dixit S, DiFiori JP, Burton M, et al. Management of patellofemoral pain syndrome. Am Fam Physician 2007;75(2):194–202.

61. Fulkerson JP. Diagnosis and treatment of patients with patellofemoral pain. Am J Sports Med 2002;30(3):447–56.

62. Post WR. Anterior knee pain: diagnosis and treatment. J Am Acad Orthop Surg 2005;13(8):534–43.

63. Macmull S, Jaiswal PK, Bentley G, et al. The role of autologous chondrocyte implantation in the treatment of symptomatic chondromalacia patellae. Int Orthop 2012;36(7):1371–7.

64. Jassim SS, Douglas SL, Haddad FS. Athletic activity after lower limb arthroplasty: a systematic review of current evidence. Bone Joint J 2014;96B(7):923–7.

65. Kettunen JA, Harilainen A, Sandelin J, et al. Knee arthroscopy and exercise versus exercise only for chronic patellofemoral pain syndrome: a randomized controlled trial. BMC Med 2007;5:38.

66. Kettunen JA, Harilainen A, Sandelin J, et al. Knee arthroscopy and exercise versus exercise only for chronic patellofemoral pain syndrome: 5-year follow-up. Br J Sports Med 2012;46(4):243–6.

67. Knoch F, Bohm T, Burgi ML, et al. Trochleaplasty for recurrent patellar dislocation in association with trochlear dysplasia. A 4- to 14-year follow-up study. J Bone Joint Surg Br 2006;88B:1331–5.

68. Schottle PB, Fucentese SF, Pfirrmann C, et al. Trochleaplasty for patellar instability due to trochlear dysplasia: a minimum 2-year clinical and radiological follow-up of 19 knees. Acta Orthop 2005;76:693–8.

69. Tecklenburg K, Feller JA, Whitehead TS, et al. Outcome of surgery for recurrent patellar dislocation based on the distance of the tibial tuberosity to the trochlear groove. J Bone Joint Surg Br 2010;92:1376–80.

70. Neumann MV, Stalder M, Schuster AJ. Reconstructive surgery for patellofemoral joint incongruency. Knee Surg Sports Traumatol Arthrosc 2014 Oct 31. [Epub ahead of print].

71. Rodriguez-Merchan EC. Evidence based conservative management of patellofemoral syndrome. Arch Bone Jt Surg 2014;2(1):4–6.

72. Crossley K, Bennell K, Green S, et al. Physical therapy for patellofemoral pain: a randomized, double-blinded, placebo-controlled trial. Am J Sports Med 2002; 30(6):857–65.

73. Dutton RA, Khadavi MJ, Fredericson M. Update on rehabilitation of patellofemoral pain. Curr Sports Med Rep 2014;13(3):172–8.

74. Frye JL, Ramey LN, Hart JM. The effects of exercise on decreasing pain and increasing function in patients with patellofemoral pain syndrome: a systematic review. Sports Health 2012;4(3):205–10.

75. Harvie D, O'Leary T, Kumar S. A systematic review of randomized controlled trials on exercise parameters in the treatment of patellofemoral pain: what works? J Multidiscip Healthc 2011;4:383–92.

76. Keays SL, Mason M, Newcombe PA. Individualized physiotherapy in the treatment of patellofemoral pain. Physiother Res Int 2014 May 22. [Epub ahead of print].

77. Lack S, Barton C, Vicenzino B, et al. Outcome predictors for conservative patellofemoral pain management: a systematic review and meta-analysis. Sports Med 2014;44(12):1703–16.

78. van Linschoten R, van Middelkoop M, Berger MY, et al. Supervised exercise therapy versus usual care for patellofemoral pain syndrome: an open label randomised controlled trial. BMJ 2009;339:b4074.

79. Rathleff MS, Roos EW, Olesen JL, et al. Early intervention for adolescents with patellofemoral pain syndrome: a pragmatic cluster randomised controlled trial. BMC Musculoskelet Disord 2012;13:9.

80. Boling MC, Bolgla LA, Mattacola CG, et al. Outcomes of a weight-bearing rehabilitation program for patients diagnosed with patellofemoral pain syndrome. Arch Phys Med Rehabil 2006;87:1428–35.

81. Cowan SM, Bennell KL, Crossley KM, et al. Physical therapy alters recruitment of the vasti in patellofemoral pain syndrome. Med Sci Sports Exerc 2002;34(12): 1879–85.

82. Earl JE, Schmitz RJ, Arnold BL. Activation of the VMO and VL during dynamic mini-squat exercises with and without isometric hip adduction. J Electromyogr Kinesiol 2001;11(6):381–6.

83. Zwerver J, Bredeweg SW, Hof AL. Biomechanical analysis of the single-leg decline squat. Br J Sports Med 2007;41:264–8.

84. Aminaka N, Gribble PA. Patellar taping, patellofemoral pain syndrome, lower extremity kinematics, and dynamic postural control. J Athl Train 2008;43(1):21–8.

85. Freedman SR, Thein Brody L, Rosenthal M, et al. Short-term effects of patellar kinesio taping on pain and hop function in patients with patellofemoral pain syndrome. Sports Health 2014;6(4):294–300.

86. Kaya D, Callaghan MJ, Ozkan H, et al. The effect of an exercise program in conjunction with short-period patellar taping on pain, electromyogram activity, and muscle strength in patellofemoral pain syndrome. Sports Health 2010;2(5):410–6.

87. Hart JM, Rothermich MA. Star excursion balance test in the evaluation of dynamic postural stability. Athletic Training & Sports Health Care 2012;4(5):201–2.

88. Callaghan MJ, Oldham JA. Electric muscle stimulation of the quadriceps in the treatment of patellofemoral pain. Arch Phys Med Rehabil 2004;85:956–62.

89. Garcia FR, Azevedo FM, Alves N, et al. Effects of electrical stimulation of vastus medialis obliquus muscle in patients with patellofemoral pain syndrome: an electromyographic analysis. Rev Bras Fisioter 2010;14(6):477–82.

90. Witvrouw E, Danneels L, van Tiggelen D, et al. Open versus closed kinetic chain exercises in patellofemoral pain: a 5-year prospective randomized study. Am J Sports Med 2004;32(5):1122–30.

91. Peters JS, Tyson NL. Proximal exercises are effective in treating patellofemoral pain syndrome: a systematic review. Int J Sports Phys Ther 2013;8(5):689–700.

92. Earl JE, Hoch AZ. A proximal strengthening program improves pain, function, and biomechanics in women with patellofemoral pain syndrome. Am J Sports Med 2011;39:154–63.

93. Nakagawa TH, Muniz TB, Baldon Rde M, et al. The effect of additional strengthening of hip abductor and lateral rotator muscles in patellofemoral pain syndrome: a randomized controlled pilot study. Clin Rehabil 2008;22:1051–60.

94. Cambridge EDJ, Sidorkewicz N, Ideda DM, et al. Progressive hip rehabilitation: the effects of resistance band placement on gluteal activation during two common exercises. Clin Biomech (Bristol, Avon) 2012;27(7):719–24.

95. Snyder KR, Earl JE, O'Connor KM, et al. Resistance training is accompanied by increases in hip strength and changes in lower extremity biomechanics during training. Clin Biomech (Bristol, Avon) 2009;24(1):26–34.
96. Hamstra-Wright KL, Huxel Bliven K. Effective exercises for targeting the gluteus medius. J Sport Rehabil 2012;21(3):296–300.
97. Lewis CL, Sahrmann SA, Moran DW. Effect of position and alteration in synergist muscle force contribution on hip forces when performing hip strengthening exercises. Clin Biomech (Bristol, Avon) 2009;24(1):35–42.
98. Kooiker L, van de Port IG, Weir A, et al. Effects of physical therapist-guided quadriceps-strengthening exercises for the treatment of patellofemoral pain syndrome: a systematic review. J Orthop Sports Phys Ther 2014;44(6):391-B1.

Supervised Rehabilitation Versus Home Exercise in the Treatment of Acute Ankle Sprains: A Systematic Review

Mark A. Feger, MEd, ATC[a], C. Collin Herb, MEd, ATC[a],
John J. Fraser, MS, PT, OCS[a,b], Neal Glaviano, MEd, ATC[a],
Jay Hertel, PhD, ATC[a,*]

KEYWORDS

- Ankle instability • Physical therapy • Therapeutic exercise

KEY POINTS

- Compared with home exercise programs, supervised rehabilitation results in less pain and subjective instability at 8 weeks after ankle sprain, but not at longer term follow-up points.
- Supervised rehabilitation results in greater gains in ankle strength and proprioception compared with home exercise at 4 months after ankle sprain.
- The incidence of recurrent ankle sprains in the 12 months after ankle sprain is equivocal between patients treated with supervised rehabilitation and home exercise.
- Only 11% of ankle sprain patients in the general population receive supervised rehabilitation within 30 days of being diagnosed with an acute ankle sprain.

Ankle sprains are the most common large joint injury incurred by competitive and recreational athletes.[1] Ankle sprains are also the most common recurrent injury seen in high school athletes.[2] Additionally, the long-term outcomes after ankle sprain are often poor. Up to 45% of patients report an incomplete recovery at 3 years after injury[3] and patients with chronic symptoms after ankle sprain report diminished self-reported function and being less physically active because of their ankle pathology.[4,5] Despite these outcomes, many individuals who incur an ankle sprain choose to not seek formal health

Disclosure Statement: The views expressed in this article are those of the authors and do not necessarily reflect the official policy or position of the Department of the Navy, Department of Defense, nor the U.S. Government.
[a] Department of Kinesiology, University of Virginia, 210 Emmet Street South, Charlottesville, VA 22904-4407, USA; [b] US Navy Medicine Professional Development Center, Bethesda, MD, USA
* Corresponding author. Department of Kinesiology, University of Virginia, 210 Emmet Street, South Charlottesville, VA 22904-4407.
E-mail address: jhertel@virginia.edu

care for this injury.[6] Among those patients who do seek treatment, there is consensus that functional treatment allowing early motion and a return to pain-free weight bearing is preferred to prolonged immobilization for mild and moderate ankle sprains,[7–9] although a period of immobilization may be preferred in severe ankle sprains.[10]

Functional treatment typically consists of protected active range of motion, stretching exercises, and neuromuscular training emphasizing balance exercises. In many organized sports settings, including professional, intercollegiate, and many interscholastic settings, these rehabilitation programs are closely supervised by athletic trainers or physical therapists. Such treatment is ubiquitous in the practice of sports medicine in these settings; however, when patients who participate in less organized athletics incur ankle sprains, they are often not referred for supervised rehabilitation. Supervised rehabilitation is the undisputed standard of care for patients participating in highly organized athletics, but is not the usual treatment in the general population. Our primary purpose was to review the best available research literature that has investigated whether clinical outcomes differ between ankle sprain patients who perform supervised rehabilitation versus unsupervised home exercise programs. Our secondary purpose was to estimate the rate of referral of ankle sprain patients to physical therapy in an effort to determine how commonly supervised rehabilitation is used in the treatment of acute ankle sprain and assess whether it is the current standard of care in the general population.

REVIEW OF RANDOMIZED, CONTROLLED TRIALS
Review Process

A systematic search of PubMed, Web of Science, CINAHL, and Medline (OVID) databases was independently performed by 3 of the co-authors (MAF, CCH, JJF) using the search terms: ankle AND (sprain OR sprains OR [ligamentous injury] OR [ligament injury]) AND ([home program] OR care OR treatment OR rehabilitation OR therapy OR physiotherapy OR training OR rehab OR management OR exercise OR intervention) NOT (deltoid OR syndesmosis OR [high ankle]). No search limit was placed on publication date, so dates ranged from the retrospective limits of each database up to September 2014. The 3 reviewers collaborated at each stage of the study selection process, with each stage progressing only after consensus was reached between reviewers (**Fig. 1**). A total of 602 studies were initially identified and 352 remained after removing duplicates. All 3 reviewers then screened for relevant studies based on title and an additional 317 studies were removed. The final 35 studies were assessed for eligibility. After screening by abstract, only 9 studies remained and only 4 of those studies[11–14] met our inclusion criteria, as described in Review Findings. The remaining 5 studies[15–19] did not meet our inclusion criteria because they were not clinical trials comparing supervised and home exercise programs for lateral ankle sprains. The 5 studies that were screened out via full text review and the 4 included studies were cross-referenced in an attempt to identify additional studies that may have been missed in our electronic search; however, no additional studies were identified.

Studies were only included if they were a randomized, controlled trial (RCT) that compared the prescription of supervised rehabilitation to unsupervised home exercise programs following an acute lateral ankle sprain. Studies were included if they analyzed any subjective patient-reported outcome (ankle sprain recurrence, pain, subjective instability, or function) or objective laboratory or clinical measures (range of motion, strength, postural control, or joint position sense). Studies were limited to clinical trials conducted on human subjects that were written in English. We did not

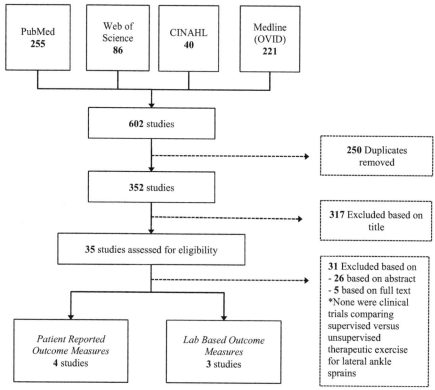

Fig. 1. Search results to identify randomized, controlled trials comparing supervised rehabilitation with unsupervised home exercises in ankle sprain patients.

exclude studies based on grade of ankle sprain or whether the ankle sprains were first or recurrent sprains.

The 4 included studies were assessed for methodological quality using the PEDro scale,[20] a 10-point scale used to assess methodological quality of original research studies. A higher PEDro value suggests a higher quality study design and methodology. Each included study was independently assessed by 2 co-authors (MF, CH) who had previous experience of using the Pedro scale. Both reviewers scored each item for each included article. If the 2 reviewers were not in consensus on an individual item, they discussed the item to reach a consensus. In the event a consensus could not be achieved between the 2 reviewers, a third co-author (JH) with extensive experience with the PEDro scale determined final score.

Patient-reported outcomes and objective measures were extracted from the selected studies. For all measures on a continuous scale, Cohen's d effect sizes[21] and associated 95% CI were calculated using the formula:

$$d = \frac{\text{Supervised Group Mean} - \text{Home Exercise Group Mean}}{\text{Home Exercise Group Standard Deviation}}$$

Additionally, to assess the effects of supervised and unsupervised rehabilitation on ankle sprain recurrence, we calculated numbers needed to treat (NNT) estimates and associated 95% CIs. Owing to the heterogeneity in treatment parameters and outcome measures of the included studies, a meta-analysis was not performed.[22]

The strength-of-recommendation taxonomy[23] was used to assess the quality and consistency of the evidence. The strength-of-recommendation taxonomy levels of evidence range from 1 (good-quality, patient-oriented evidence) to 2 (limited-quality, patient-oriented evidence) to 3 (other evidence), and the strength of recommendations range from A (recommendation is based on consistent and good-quality, patient-oriented evidence) to B (inconsistent or limited-quality, patient-oriented evidence), to C (evidence other than patient-oriented evidence).[23]

Review Findings

Our search strategy yielded 4 RCTs[11-14] that compared supervised versus unsupervised rehabilitation in ankle sprain patients (**Table 1**). Details of the methodological quality assessment are provided in **Table 2**. PEDro scores for the included studies ranged from 5 to 8. The most common PEDro items that were not met were related to blinding of subjects and clinicians, but because of the nature of the study interventions it is impossible to blind the subjects or treating clinicians as to whether they received supervised rehabilitation or home exercise. Thus, the highest feasible PEDro score that a study could receive should be considered 8 rather than 10. It must be noted that 2 of the included studies[13,14] consisted mostly of the same patients, but with follow-up measures reported at different time points.

Patient self-reported outcomes

Effect size point estimates and the associated 95% CIs for comparisons of patient self-reported outcomes are illustrated in **Figs. 2** and **3**. There was a trend toward the supervised rehabilitation groups reporting less pain and less subjective instability than the home exercise groups at 8-week follow-up; however, the results between groups were equivocal at the 3- and 12-month follow-up assessments. Both treatment groups demonstrated improvements in pain, subjective instability, and subjective recovery across the course of the follow-up periods.

Clinical and laboratory measure outcomes

For measures of range of motion, strength, postural control, and joint position sense, effect size point estimates and associated 95% CIs are shown in **Fig. 4**. At the 6-week follow-up, the supervised rehabilitation group demonstrated greater dorsiflexion strength, but less eversion strength than the home exercise group. All other comparisons at 6-week follow-up were equivocal between groups. Likewise at 3-month follow-up, there was no conclusive difference in dorsiflexion range of motion between groups. However, at the 4-month follow-up, the supervised rehabilitation group showed large improvements in joint position sense and dorsiflexion, plantar flexion, and eversion strength compared with the home exercise group. In contrast, the home exercise group reported large improvements in postural control compared with the supervised rehabilitation group at 4-month follow-up.

Ankle sprain recurrence

Results of the NNT analysis are illustrated in **Fig. 5**. Holme and colleagues[12] revealed a substantial reduction in ankle sprain recurrence at 12-month follow-up in the supervised rehabilitation group compared with the unsupervised group with an NNT estimate of 5 (95% CI, 5–18). However, the van Rijn and colleagues[13,14] studies demonstrated no conclusive difference, as indicated by the extremely wide CIs that crossed infinity, in recurrent sprains between the 2 groups at the 8-week, 12-week, or 12-month follow-up assessments. Additionally, ankle sprain severity did not seem to influence conclusively the results of the interventions on ankle sprain recurrence (**Fig. 6**).

Grading the evidence

Compared with lateral ankle sprain patients performing unsupervised home exercise programs, patients receiving supervised rehabilitation programs had (1) less pain and subjective instability at intermediate follow-up (8 weeks after injury), but no differences in self-reported outcomes at longer follow-up periods (3 and 12 months after injury), (2) greater gains in ankle strength and joint position sense, but worse postural control, at the 4-month follow-up, and (3) inconclusive results regarding prevention of recurrent ankle sprains in the 12 months after injury. We conclude that a strength-of-recommendation taxonomy grade of 2B for these findings based on the preponderance of inconsistent or limited quality, patient-oriented evidence across the included studies.

SUPERVISED REHABILITATION REFERRAL PATTERNS

To quantify the frequency at which patients who are diagnosed with a lateral ankle sprain underwent supervised rehabilitation, we queried the PearlDiver Patient Record Database (PearlDiver Inc, Fort Wayne, IN). This commercially available database contains patient data from private insurance companies and does not include uninsured patients or those insured via Medicare or Medicaid. The database contains more than 1.1 billion patient records on more than 30 million individual patients records between 2007 and 2011. The database can be used to identify *International Classification of Disease, Ninth Revision* (ICD-9) codes and Current Procedural Terminology (CPT) codes.

The database was queried for patients who had been diagnosed with ICD-9 codes for lateral ankle sprains but not medial ankle sprains with the following algorithm ([845.00 -Unspecified ankle sprain] OR [845.02 – calcaneofibular ligament sprain] NOT [845.01 – deltoid ligament sprain]). We then queried these patients for those who had an associated CPT code for therapeutic exercise (97110, 97112, 97530, or 97116) or manual therapy (97140) within 1 month of the diagnosis of a lateral ankle sprain. CPT codes for therapeutic exercise included range of motion, strength, balance training, gait training, and functional exercises, whereas manual therapy codes included joint mobilizations and manipulations.

Referral patterns for supervised rehabilitation within 30 days of ankle sprain diagnosis are illustrated in **Fig. 7**. Of the 825,718 patients diagnosed with a lateral ankle sprain, only 89,539 (11%) had an associated billing code for supervised rehabilitation or manual therapy within 30 days of their ankle sprain diagnosis. For those receiving supervised rehabilitation, the most common therapeutic exercise or manual therapy physical therapy treatments billed for were strength and range of motion (97% of all supervised rehabilitation patients), joint mobilization or manipulation (62%), balance or postural control (32%), functional exercise (20%), and gait training (4%).

CLINICAL RECOMMENDATIONS

Our review of RCTs revealed that, compared with unsupervised home exercise programs, supervised rehabilitation programs resulted in (1) less pain and subjective instability at intermediate follow-up (8 weeks after injury), but no differences in self-reported outcomes at longer follow-up periods (3 and 12 months after injury), (2) greater gains in ankle strength and joint position sense, but worse postural control, at the 4-month follow-up, and (3) inconclusive results regarding prevention of

Table 1
Characteristics of the 4 randomized, controlled trials (RCTs) comparing supervised rehabilitation and unsupervised home exercise programs in patients recovering from acute ankle sprains

Author, Year, Design	Sample Population	Inclusion Criteria	Groups/Intervention	Assessment Time Points and Outcomes
van Rijn et al,[13] 2007, RCT	Supervised (n = 49): 21 female, 28 male Age: 37.0 ± 11.9 y 4.8 d between injury and baseline Unsupervised (n = 53): 22 female, 31 male Age: 37.0 ± 11.9 y 4.6 d between injury and baseline	Setting: Physician office or emergency department Lateral ankle sprain treated within 1 wk of injury 18–60 y of age	Supervised (nine 30-min treatment sessions that included balance, walking, running and jump exercises over 3 mo) Unsupervised (advice for early mobilization/weight bearing and home exercises with written instructions)	3 mo, and 1 y post injury Subjective recovery Report of recurrence of sprain 3 mo Dorsiflexion range of motion
van Rijn et al,[14] 2009, subgroup analysis of 2007 RCT	**Ankle function score ≤40 (n = 56)** Supervised (n = 28): 14 female, 14 male Age: 39.3 ± 12.7 y Unsupervised (n = 28): 12 female, 16 male Age: 38.8 ± 13.3 y **Ankle function score >40 (n = 46)** Supervised (n = 21): 7 female, 14 male Age: 34.0 ± 10.4 y Unsupervised (n = 25): 11 female, 14 male Age: 35.0 ± 10.0 y	Setting: Physician office or emergency department Lateral ankle sprain treated within 1 wk of injury 18–60 y of age	Supervised (nine 30-min treatment sessions that included balance, walking, running and jump exercises over 3 mo) Unsupervised (advice for early mobilization/weight bearing and home exercises with written instructions)	8 wk and 1 y post injury Subjective recovery Report of recurrence of sprain Self-reports of pain and instability

Study	Subjects	Setting	Intervention	Outcomes
Basset & Prapavessis,[11] 2007, prospective RCT	Supervised (n = 25): 11 female, 14 male, Age: 29.3 ± 13.8 y; Unsupervised (n = 22): 8 female, 14 male, Age: 30.9 ± 11.0 y	Setting: Physical therapy clinics; First time or recurrent lateral ankle sprain	Three-phase intervention protocol progressed based on severity and progress of recovery (acute, mobilizing, strengthening). Supervised: Active range of motion, stretching, strengthening, taping/strapping, balance training and dynamic and functional training. Unsupervised: 1 visit for instruction at the transition of each treatment phase. Patients provided an instructional booklet, Tubigrip, Thera-band resistance bands, and wobble boards.	Baseline and immediately after intervention. Ankle function: Lower Limb Task Questionnaire; Motor Activity Scale
Holme et al,[12] 1999, prospective RCT	Supervised (n = 29): 12 female, 17 male, Age: 25.5 ± 3.8 y; Unsupervised (n = 42): 15 female, 27 male, Age: 27.4 ± 4.6 y	Emergency department; Acute lateral ankle sprain	Supervised: Education on early ankle mobilization, strength, mobility, and balance (eyes open and closed) with a balance board. Group physical therapy 2 h/wk. Additional exercises included figure 8 running, balance with ball toss, and positional balance on inside and the outside of the foot. Unsupervised: Education on early ankle mobilization, strength, mobility, and balance (eyes open and closed) with a balance board. Patient progression based on feelings of improvement.	6 wk and 4 mo after intervention. Compared injured with uninjured limbs in each group. Dorsiflexion, plantarflexion, eversion, inversion strength; Postural sway; Position sense

Table 2
PEDro scoring of methodological quality of 4 randomized, controlled trials that compared supervised rehabilitation and unsupervised home exercise programs in patients recovering from acute ankle sprains

	van Rijn et al,[13] 2007	van Rijn et al,[14] 2009	Bassett & Prapavessis,[11] 2007	Holme et al,[12] 1999
Eligibility criteria?	Y	Y	Y	Y
Random allocation?	Y	Y	Y	Y
Allocation concealed?	Y	Y	Y	Y
Groups similar?	Y	Y	Y	N
Subject blinding?	N	N	N	N
Therapist blinding?	N	N	N	N
Assessor blinding?	Y	Y	N	N
85% subjects completed?	Y	Y	Y	N
Allocation maintained or intention to treat?	Y	N	Y	Y
Between-group statistical comparisons?	Y	Y	Y	Y
Point and variability measures reported?	Y	Y	Y	Y
PEDro Score	8/10	7/10	7/10	5/10

Abbreviations: N, No; Y, yes.

recurrent ankle sprains in the 12 months after injury. It must be emphasized that these conclusions are drawn from studies done primarily in community settings and not competitive sports medicine settings. Regardless, these results are likely to be seen as surprising to rehabilitation clinicians who work in competitive sports medicine settings, where the supervised treatment and rehabilitation of patients with ankle sprains is viewed as the standard of care.

Supervised rehabilitation was found to improve subjective outcomes, specifically less pain and feelings of subjective instability, than unsupervised home exercise programs at 8 weeks of follow-up but not at later time points. Do improved patient reported outcomes in the short -term, but equivocal outcomes in the long term, justify the added cost and time associated with supervised rehabilitation? This is a question that is debatable and is likely to have different responses depending on who is answering the question. Patients are likely to favor supervised treatment, at least temporarily, if it results in them feeling better, even if only in the short term. Rehabilitation clinicians are also likely to favor supervised treatment because it provides a level of validation for the health care they are providing. Individuals responsible for making payment decisions, such as those responsible for third-party reimbursement, may be less swayed by the importance of short-term, but not long-term, improvements seen in ankle sprain patients treated with supervised rehabilitation rather than home exercise programs. Our review did not address cost–benefit or the cost effectiveness of these 2 treatment approaches, but this is an area that is ripe for further study.

There were conflicting results in terms of prevention of recurrent ankle sprains across the 3 studies[12–14] that tracked recurrence. The Holme and colleagues[12] study showed conclusive prevention of recurrent sprains in the 12 months after initial injury for the supervised rehabilitation group compared with the unsupervised group,

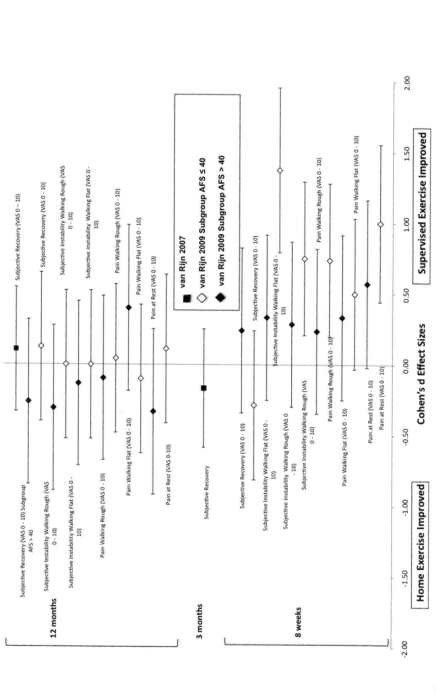

Fig. 2. Effect sizes and 95% CIs of patient self-reported outcome measures comparing supervised rehabilitation with home exercise in ankle sprain patients. VAS, visual analog scale.

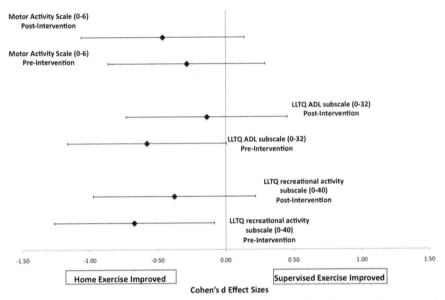

Fig. 3. Effect sizes and 95% CIs of outcome measures for the Bassett and colleagues study comparing the supervised rehabilitation and home exercise groups at before and after the intervention. The manner in which the data were presented in the original article prevented the same between group calculations being made as were performed in **Fig. 2**. ADL, activities of daily living; LLTQ, lower limb task questionnaire.

whereas the 2 van Rijn and colleagues[13,14] studies did not show group differences in recurrent ankle sprains. The reason for this disparity is unclear. Holme and colleagues[12] documented strength and joint position sense gains in the supervised rehabilitation group at 4 months of follow-up, whereas van Rijn and colleagues[13,14] did not track any neuromuscular outcomes. It is possible that the structure of the supervised rehabilitation programs across studies influenced the disparate outcomes.

The American Physical Therapy Association has recently published clinical practice guidelines for the management of patients with ankle sprains.[24] Their recommended treatments include the encouragement of early weight bearing with necessary external ankle support, the use of cryotherapy in the acute phase of recovery, manual therapy to initially assist with pain control and edema reduction, mobilization and manipulation techniques to aid in the restoration of range of motion, and progressive functional exercises, including balance training.[24] It seems that the RCTs in our review mostly followed the principles outlined in the current clinical practice guidelines, although the explicit use of manual therapy is not addressed in the protocols of any these studies.

Much of the recent scholarship in the area of supervised rehabilitation for lateral ankle injuries has been related to the treatment of patients with chronic ankle instability (CAI). Donovan and Hertel[25] presented a paradigm for treating patients with CAI that utilized an "assess–treat–reassess" framework in the multiple areas of functional impairments including range of motion (both osteokinematic and arthrokinematic), strength, balance, and functional movements, such as walking, running, cutting, and landing. This paradigm emphasized individualized treatment approaches based on patient-specific deficits. Such an approach is only feasible in a supervised

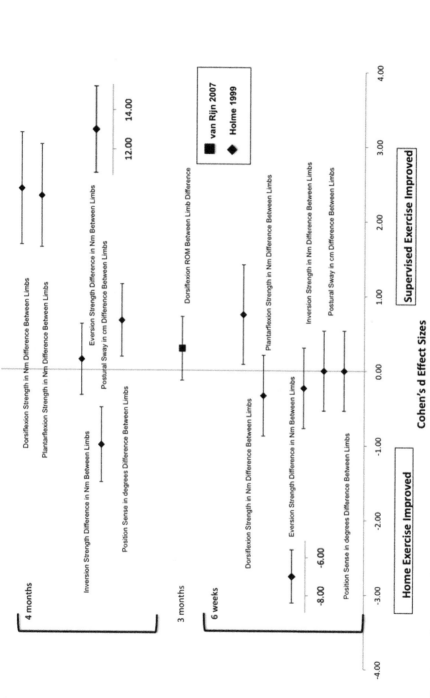

Fig. 4. Effect sizes and 95% CIs of laboratory measures of strength, postural control, and joint position sense comparing supervised rehabilitation to home exercise in ankle sprain patients. Note the condensed scales for extremely large CIs on both the right and left sides of the graph. Nm, Newton meters; ROM, range of motion.

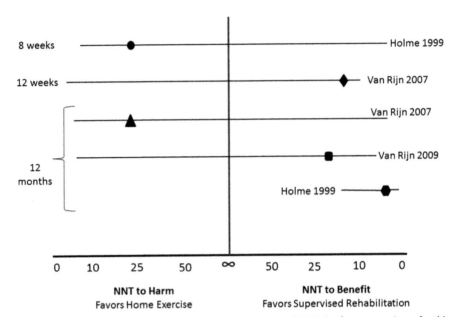

Fig. 5. Numbers needed to treat (NNT) point estimates and 95% CIs for prevention of ankle sprain recurrence in supervised rehabilitation versus home exercise groups.

rehabilitation setting and not in a home exercise setting. Likewise, McKeon and colleagues[26] emphasized the utility of objective performance criteria when progressing CAI patients to more advanced levels of therapeutic exercise during supervised rehabilitation. Again, this approach is less feasible in a home exercise setting. Our

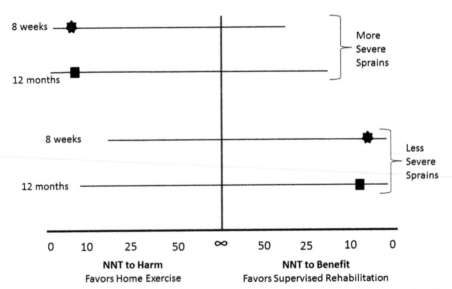

Fig. 6. Numbers needed to treat (NNT) point estimates and 95% CIs for prevention of ankle sprain recurrence in the supervised rehabilitation versus home exercise groups in the subgroups defined as having more or less severe ankle sprains in the van Rijn et al. (2009) study.

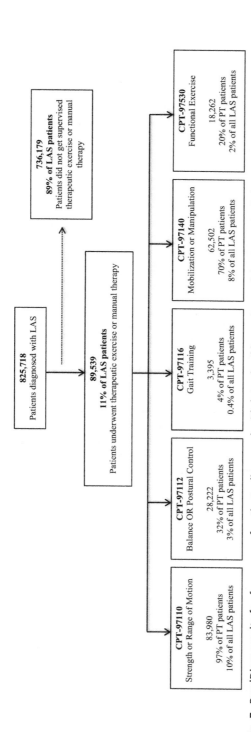

Fig. 7. PearlDiver results for frequency of patients diagnosed with lateral ankle sprain receiving supervised therapeutic exercise or manual therapy Current Procedural Terminology (CPT) codes within 30 days of ankle sprain diagnosis. LAS, lateral ankle sprain; PT, physical therapy (operationally defined as therapeutic exercise or manual therapy).

recommendation is that an acute ankle sprain rehabilitation paradigm using the "assess–treat–reassess" model across multiple areas of functional impairments be combined with the use of objective therapeutic exercise progression criteria be subjected to rigorous evaluation against home exercise in a RCT.

Another area of rehabilitation that is difficult to administer in a home exercise treatment regimen is manual therapy. Although some manual therapy techniques can be performed via self-mobilizations,[27] joint mobilizations and manipulations at the ankle are typically performed by skilled rehabilitation clinicians. There is considerable evidence of the effectiveness of joint mobilizations and manipulations in reducing pain and increasing ankle motion in patients recovering from ankle sprains.[28–31] Interestingly, none of the 4 RCTs that we reviewed stated explicitly whether joint mobilizations or manipulations were included in the supervised rehabilitation regimens that were employed. However, a recent study by Cleland and colleagues[16] demonstrated that ankle sprain patients receiving manual therapy and performing home exercise had greater improvements in self-reported function at 4-week and 6-month follow-up visits than patients only performing home exercise. Although this demonstrates the efficacy of manual therapy, it does not assess whether supervised rehabilitation and manual therapy are better than home exercise alone. Given the research evidence demonstrating the effectiveness of manual therapy in the treatment of ankle sprain patients, a study investigating the effects of supervised rehabilitation with manual therapy in comparison with manual therapy with home exercise and to home exercise alone is needed to fully understand the effects of supervised rehabilitation.

Completion of unsupervised home exercise is associated with better outcomes than not performing any therapeutic exercise after ankle sprain.[18] Wester and colleagues[18] reported a significant reduction in recurrent ankle sprains at the 8-month follow-up assessment in a group of ankle sprain patients who performed 15 minutes of wobble board training daily for 12 weeks compared with a group that only received standardized instructions after their ankle sprain diagnosis. The NNT from this study was previously reported as 5 (95% CI, 3–17), indicating a conclusive reduction in ankle sprain recurrence in group completing home exercise compared with the group not performing any therapeutic exercise.[32] Likewise, Hupperets and colleagues[17] reported that athletes, defined as active sports participants aged 12 to 70, performing an 8-week program of unsupervised balance board exercises (3 days per week for up to 30 minutes per day) had significantly less recurrent ankle sprains than athletes not performing any therapeutic exercises. An NNT of 9 (no CI provided) was reported along with a relative risk of recurrent sprain within 12 months of 0.63 (95% CI, 0.45–0.88), favoring the home exercise group. Collectively, these results clearly show the benefit of home exercise programs versus no exercise program in the prevention of recurrent ankle sprains.

An issue that is critical with therapeutic exercise, whether performed as part of supervised rehabilitation or a home exercise program, is compliance. Several recent studies have reported low compliance levels with home exercise programs. Hupperets and colleagues[17] reported that 23% of their unsupervised exercise group reported to be fully compliant, 29% were partially compliant, and 35% were not compliant with their 8-week intervention. The compliance of the remaining 13% was unknown because of failure of subjects to complete the compliance questionnaire. Similarly, in a study[33] comparing ankle bracing, unsupervised therapeutic exercise, and a combination of bracing and exercise on ankle sprain recurrence, full compliance was reported by 45% of the exercise group, 23% of the bracing group, and 28% in the combination group. Although compliance rates have not been reported commonly in supervised rehabilitation groups, it is reasonable to assume that they are higher than for unsupervised exercise groups.

Interestingly, the results of the Janssen and colleagues[33] study indicated that bracing was superior at preventing recurrent ankle sprains compared with the unsupervised exercise and there was not an additive prevention effect of combining bracing with unsupervised therapeutic exercise. This study supports other recent large RCTs that have identified bracing as having a significant effect on ankle sprain prevention in competitive athletes.[34,35]

In the United States, the use of supervised rehabilitation in the treatment of acute ankle sprains in competitive sports medicine settings is inescapable and largely unquestioned. In fact, it is common that competitive athletes undergo supervised rehabilitation from an athletic trainer or sports physical therapist several times per day while recovering from an acute ankle sprain. We were, therefore, surprised to find that only 11% of ankle sprain patients in the general population had supervised rehabilitation codes filed with their health insurance companies within 30 days of their ankle sprain diagnosis. This begs the question as to why there are so few patients with ankle sprains being referred for supervised rehabilitation. Is it, as demonstrated in our review (see **Figs. 2–6**), because of a lack of clear evidence supporting the use of supervised rehabilitation in the treatment of ankle sprains? Or, perhaps, is there an underappreciation of the long-term, negative outcomes associated with ankle sprains? This underappreciation could be by patients, primary care clinicians making the majority of the initial ankle sprain diagnoses, or both. Another possibility is that many patients are seeking initial care with the explicit goal of ruling out a fracture and they are not interested in completing rehabilitation once they receive a diagnosis of ankle sprain. Issues of the cost of supervised rehabilitation services may also play a role, as could ankle sprain severity. Further research is necessary to explore the reasons for the surprisingly low referral rates of acute ankle sprain patients for supervised rehabilitation.

We were surprised that there were just 4 RCTs comparing the effects of supervised rehabilitation with home exercise programs in patients with an acute ankle sprain. Additionally, there were no RCTs identified that compared these treatments in CAI patients. There is a clear need in this area for additional RCTs with larger sample sizes, the use of consistent subjective and objective outcome measures, and longer follow-up periods. Our recommendations, based on our review, are only generalizable to the general population and not to competitive sports medicine settings. It is unclear whether the results found here would be replicated in the competitive sports medicine settings where aggressive supervised rehabilitation of acute ankle sprains is the norm. It is necessary for future investigators to evaluate whether the more aggressive supervised rehabilitation treatments common in competitive sports medicine settings could be used to improve clinical outcomes in the general population, and whether the less time-consuming and less expensive home exercise approaches, shown to be largely equivocal to supervised rehabilitation in the general population, could be applied to the competitive sports medicine settings without compromising outcomes. The only way to conclusively answer these questions is by performing well-designed clinical trials.

Our clinical recommendations are that supervised rehabilitation results in short-term benefits in self-reported measures of patient function and objective measures of neuromuscular performance that are likely to be important to patients. Despite the lack of consistent improvements at the 1-year follow-up with supervised rehabilitation compared with unsupervised home exercise, we recommend the use of supervised rehabilitation in the treatment of acute ankle sprains because of the improved short-term outcomes. Additionally, if supervised rehabilitation is not feasible for a patient, a home exercise program is strongly recommended. The CAI literature supports the use of progressive, impairment-based supervised rehabilitation and there is a clear need to study this model in the acute ankle sprain population.[25,26,36] Last, we recommend the use prophylactic ankle bracing to aid in the prevention of recurrent ankle sprains.[33–35]

SUMMARY

The best research evidence demonstrated that supervised rehabilitation programs resulted in (1) less pain and subjective instability at intermediate follow-up (8 weeks after injury), but no differences in self-reported outcomes at longer follow-up periods (3 and 12 months after injury), (2) greater gains in ankle strength and joint position sense, but worse postural control, at the 4-month follow-up, and (3) inconclusive results regarding prevention of recurrent ankle sprains at 12 months after injury. A surprisingly small number of patients (11%) in the general population diagnosed with acute ankle sprains undergo supervised rehabilitation. There is a clear disconnect between how patients with ankle sprains are treated in competitive sports medicine settings compared with the general population.

REFERENCES

1. Hootman JM, Dick R, Agel J. Epidemiology of collegiate injuries for 15 sports: summary and recommendations for injury prevention initiatives. J Athl Train 2007;42(2):311–9.
2. Swenson DM, Yard EE, Fields SK, et al. Patterns of recurrent injuries among US high school athletes, 2005–2008. Am J Sports Med 2009;37(8):1586–93.
3. van Rijn RM, van Os AG, Bernsen RM, et al. What is the clinical course of acute ankle sprains? A systematic literature review. Am J Med 2008;121(4):324–31.
4. Anandacoomarasamy A, Barnsley L. Long term outcomes of inversion ankle injuries. Br J Sports Med 2005;39(3):e14.
5. Verhagen R, De Keizer G, Van Dijk C. Long-term follow-up of inversion trauma of the ankle. Arch Orthop Trauma Surg 1995;114(2):92–6.
6. McKay GD, Goldie PA, Payne WR, et al. Ankle injuries in basketball: Injury rate and risk factors. Br J Sports Med 2001;35(2):103–8.
7. Bleakley CM, O'Connor SR, Tully MA, et al. Effect of accelerated rehabilitation on function after ankle sprain: randomised controlled trial. BMJ 2010;340:c1964.
8. Eiff MP, Smith AT, Smith GE. Early mobilization versus immobilization in the treatment of lateral ankle sprains. Am J Sports Med 1994;22(1):83–8.
9. Jones MH, Amendola AS. Acute treatment of inversion ankle sprains: immobilization versus functional treatment. Clin Orthop Relat Res 2007;455:169–72.
10. Lamb SE, Marsh J, Hutton JL, et al. Mechanical supports for acute, severe ankle sprain: a pragmatic, multicentre, randomised controlled trial. Lancet 2009; 373(9663):575–81.
11. Bassett SF, Prapavessis H. Home-based physical therapy intervention with adherence-enhancing strategies versus clinic-based management for patients with ankle sprains. Phys Ther 2007;87(9):1132–43.
12. Holme E, Magnusson S, Becher K, et al. The effect of supervised rehabilitation on strength, postural sway, position sense and re-injury risk after acute ankle ligament sprain. Scand J Med Sci Sports 1999;9(2):104–9.
13. van Rijn RM, van Os AG, Kleinrensink G, et al. Supervised exercises for adults with acute lateral ankle sprain: a randomised controlled trial. Br J Gen Pract 2007;57(543):793–800.

14. van Rijn RM, van Heest JA, van der Wees P, et al. Some benefit from physiotherapy intervention in the subgroup of patients with severe ankle sprain as determined by the ankle function score: a randomised trial. Aust J Physiother 2009;55(2):107–13.
15. Beynnon BD, Renstrom PA, Haugh L, et al. A prospective, randomized clinical investigation of the treatment of first-time ankle sprains. Am J Sports Med 2006;34(9):1401–12.
16. Cleland JA, Mintken P, McDevitt A, et al. Manual physical therapy and exercise versus supervised home exercise in the management of patients with inversion ankle sprain: a multicenter randomized clinical trial. J Orthop Sports Phys Ther 2013;43(7):443–55.
17. Hupperets MD, Verhagen EA, van Mechelen W. Effect of unsupervised home based proprioceptive training on recurrences of ankle sprain: randomised controlled trial. BMJ 2009;339:b2684.
18. Wester JU, Jespersen SM, Nielsen KD, et al. Wobble board training after partial sprains of the lateral ligaments of the ankle: a prospective randomized study. J Orthop Sports Phys Ther 1996;23(5):332–6.
19. Christakou A, Zervas Y, Lavallee D. The adjunctive role of imagery on the functional rehabilitation of a grade II ankle sprain. Hum Mov Sci 2007;26(1):141–54.
20. Maher CG, Sherrington C, Herbert RD, et al. Reliability of the PEDro scale for rating quality of randomized controlled trials. Phys Ther 2003;83(8):713–21.
21. Cohen J. Statistical power analysis for the behavioral sciences. New York: Routledge; 1988.
22. Israel H, Richter RR. A guide to understanding meta-analysis. J Orthop Sports Phys Ther 2011;41(7):496–504.
23. Ebell MH, Siwek J, Weiss BD, et al. Strength of recommendation taxonomy (SORT): a patient-centered approach to grading evidence in the medical literature. J Am Board Fam Pract 2004;17(1):59–67.
24. Martin RL, Davenport TE, Paulseth S, et al. Ankle stability and movement coordination impairments: ankle ligament sprains: clinical practice guidelines linked to the international classification of functioning, disability and health from the orthopaedic section of the American Physical Therapy Association. J Orthop Sports Phys Ther 2013;43(9):A1–40.
25. Donovan L, Hertel J. A new paradigm for rehabilitation of patients with chronic ankle instability. Phys Sportsmed 2012;40(4):41–51.
26. McKeon P, Ingersoll C, Kerrigan DC, et al. Balance training improves function and postural control in those with chronic ankle instability. Med Sci Sports Exerc 2008; 40(10):1810.
27. Johnson KD, Grindstaff TL. Thoracic region self-mobilization: a clinical suggestion. Int J Sports Phys Ther 2012;7(2):252–6.
28. Green T, Refshauge K, Crosbie J, et al. A randomized controlled trial of a passive accessory joint mobilization on acute ankle inversion sprains. Phys Ther 2001; 81(4):984–94.
29. Loudon JK, Reiman MP, Sylvain J. The efficacy of manual joint mobilisation/manipulation in treatment of lateral ankle sprains: a systematic review. Br J Sports Med 2014;48(5):365–70.
30. Whitman JM, Cleland JA, Mintken P, et al. Predicting short-term response to thrust and nonthrust manipulation and exercise in patients post inversion ankle sprain. J Orthop Sports Phys Ther 2009;39(3):188–200.
31. van der Wees PJ, Lenssen AF, Hendriks EJ, et al. Effectiveness of exercise therapy and manual mobilisation in acute ankle sprain and functional instability: a systematic review. Aust J Physiother 2006;52(1):27–37.

32. McKeon PO, Hertel J. Systematic review of postural control and lateral ankle instability, part II: is balance training clinically effective? J Athl Train 2008;43(3): 305–15.
33. Janssen KW, van Mechelen W, Verhagen EA. Bracing superior to neuromuscular training for the prevention of self-reported recurrent ankle sprains: a three-arm randomised controlled trial. Br J Sports Med 2014;48(16):1235–9.
34. McGuine TA, Brooks A, Hetzel S. The effect of lace-up ankle braces on injury rates in high school basketball players. Am J Sports Med 2011;39(9):1840–8.
35. McGuine TA, Hetzel S, Wilson J, et al. The effect of lace-up ankle braces on injury rates in high school football players. Am J Sports Med 2012;40(1):49–57.
36. Hale SA, Hertel J, Olmsted-Kramer LC. The effect of a 4-week comprehensive rehabilitation program on postural control and lower extremity function in individuals with chronic ankle instability. J Orthop Sports Phys Ther 2007;37(6): 303–11.

Freeing the Foot

Integrating the Foot Core System into Rehabilitation for Lower Extremity Injuries

Patrick O. McKeon, PhD, ATC, CSCS[a],*, François Fourchet, PT, PhD[b]

KEYWORDS

- Foot control • Dynamic systems • Neuromuscular electrostimulation
- Overuse injury • Muscle training

KEY POINTS

- The foot core system is the integration of active, passive, and neural structures within the foot to provide dynamic foot control during functional activities.
- Lower extremity overuse injuries may be the result of a loss or restriction within one of the subsystems of the foot core, which results in increased stress on the remaining structures.
- The intrinsic foot muscles provide sensory and motor contributions to the foot core system and their dysfunction may contribute to the development of lower extremity overuse injuries.
- Training the foot muscles through a progression of isolation to integration provides a means to increase the functional variability of the foot core system in dynamic foot control.
- Neuromuscular electrostimulation of the intrinsic foot muscles provides a means of isolating these muscles for patient education and enhanced performance.

INTRODUCTION

Dynamic foot control arises from the complex interaction between active and passive structures, and the corresponding orchestration of sensory and motor information to control the configuration of the bones within the foot.[1] The unique shape and alignment of the tarsals and metatarsals coalesce into the longitudinal and transverse arches with ligamentous support from the long and short plantar ligaments, the plantar calcaneonavicular ligament, and the plantar aponeurosis.[2,3] These passive structures are also supported dynamically through the tendons of the extrinsic foot muscles and

Disclosure Statement: The authors have agreed on all content associated with this article. The authors report no conflicts of interest with any of the material presented in this article.
[a] Department of Exercise and Sport Sciences, Ithaca College, 953 Danby Road, Ithaca, NY 14850, USA; [b] Department of Physiotherapy, Hôpital La Tour Réseau de Soins, 3 Avenue J-D Maillard, Meyrin, Geneva 1217, Switzerland
* Corresponding author.
E-mail address: pmckeon@ithaca.edu

Clin Sports Med 34 (2015) 347–361
http://dx.doi.org/10.1016/j.csm.2014.12.002
0278-5919/15/$ – see front matter © 2015 Elsevier Inc. All rights reserved.

sportsmed.theclinics.com

the intrinsic foot muscles.[4] The intrinsic foot muscles are those that have origin and insertion sites within the foot. The extrinsic foot muscles are those whose muscle bellies reside proximal to the foot, but tendons directly insert into the bones and ligaments. These muscles are considered to be the prime movers of foot function, whereas the intrinsic foot muscles have typically been thought to play more of a supporting role in dynamic foot control.[5] The passive and active structures work together producing a unique ability of the foot to absorb and propel the body using the resultant forces from the foot-ground interaction.[1]

A major structure within the foot that integrates the passive and active contributions is the plantar aponeurosis.[6] Its primary function is to provide rigid support of the arches during the propulsion phase of gait, referred to as the windlass mechanism,[3] which transitions the foot from absorption to propulsion demands during stance. Although this structure and mechanism are essential for the foot, the passive nature of the plantar aponeurosis makes it difficult to detect deformation and respond to foot deformation demands. The tendons of the extrinsic foot muscles also control deformation longitudinally and rotationally during absorption. When looking at the alignments of the plantar intrinsic foot muscles, it is apparent that these muscles must provide redundancy in function to the plantar aponeurosis and the extrinsic muscle tendons providing resistance to medial arch deformation in a similar fashion, but their muscle bellies are directly aligned with the pattern of foot deformation.[1]

According to the dynamic systems theory of sensorimotor control,[7] the sensorimotor system is composed of multiple interacting components that can be organized in a variety of ways to accomplish movement goals. Within the sensorimotor system, sensory information tunes motor output and motor output tunes the subsequent change in sensory information. The foot has multiple interacting systems of passive, active, and neural components, which are integrated into the foot core system (**Fig. 1**).[1] The unique interactions of passive subsystem (eg, ligaments, plantar aponeurosis) and active subsystem (extrinsic and intrinsic foot muscles) with the

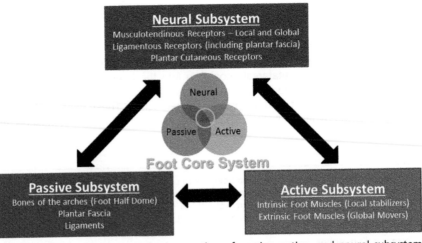

Fig. 1. The foot core system is the integration of passive, active, and neural subsystems, which provide functional variability in adapting to changing task and environmental demands during functional activities. (*From* McKeon PO, Hertel J, Bramble D, et al. The foot core system: a new paradigm for understanding intrinsic foot muscle function. Br J Sports Med 2014 Mar 21. http://dx.doi.org/10.1136/bjsports-2013-092690. [Epub ahead of print].)

neural subsystem (sensory information and motor output) within the foot core allow the foot great adaptability in that multiple degrees of freedom can be used to accomplish the movement goals of absorption and propulsion.[1] This ensures that no one degree of freedom within any of the subsystems is stressed to a greater extent than any other and is referred to as functional variability.[7,8] However, if there is a loss of degrees of freedom within the system, the reduction in functional variability may result in progressive damage of tissues beyond their ability to repair and adapt.[9] This lines up well with the description of overuse factors in the development of such conditions as plantar fasciitis,[10] medial tibial stress syndrome,[11] and stress fractures of the foot.

When examining the literature associated with rehabilitation for overabsorption types of injuries, evidence for the function of the intrinsic foot muscles and targeting improvement in their function through intervention is very minimal. Rather, the trend in the evidence focuses on the support of either the passive subsystem through foot orthotics[12–14] reducing symptoms or targeting enhanced function of the extrinsic foot muscles to limit foot deformation.[11,14,15] Both intervention strategies have some fairly consistent evidence to support their effectiveness, but training the intrinsic foot muscles and integrating them back into the foot core system to promote enhanced foot control may be a crucial missing link for the treatment of these types of overuse lower extremity conditions. This article provides a brief overview of plantar intrinsic foot muscle function within the foot core system, and a progression for isolating these muscles in rehabilitation and promoting a reintegration of these muscles with the passive, active, and neural subsystems of the foot core.

THE FUNCTIONS AND CONTRIBUTIONS OF THE INTRINSIC FOOT MUSCLES

There are plantar and dorsal muscles within the foot. There is little evidence about the dorsal intrinsic foot muscles and their role in foot function. However, this does not mean they do not play a vital role and further research is needed to elucidate their contributions to the foot core. Much more commonly investigated are the plantar intrinsic foot muscles, which consist of four layers of muscles deep to the plantar aponeurosis. The first two layers have muscle configurations that align with the medial and lateral longitudinal arches of the foot, whereas the deeper layers align more so with the anterior and posterior transverse arches.[1] The predominant role of these muscles in foot function has traditionally been viewed within the active subsystem as stabilizers rather than within the neural subsystem as deformation sensors. For this reason, most evidence concerned with these muscles is associated with their role as foot stabilizers rather than foot sensors. Within this functional role, there is controversial evidence as to their contribution to foot stability within the foot core system. However, there does seem to be a pattern that emerges across the evidence.

Fatigue or Dysfunction of the Plantar Intrinsic Foot Muscles Results in Impaired Foot Posture

Fatigue or dysfunction of the plantar intrinsic foot muscles in healthy individuals produces a subtle change in foot posture, namely an increase in navicular drop. Headlee and colleagues[16] found that after fatiguing the intrinsic foot muscles of healthy individuals through repeated isolated contractions, navicular drop increased. Fiolkowski and colleagues[17] conducted a study where the activity of the plantar intrinsic foot muscles was reduced via tibial nerve block in a cohort of healthy young men. They observed that the tibial nerve block produced a decrease in abductor hallucis activity and a concomitant increase in navicular drop. In a further study using the tibial nerve block protocol, Fiolkowski and colleagues[18] also found reduced leg muscle stiffness during a hopping task in the presence of reduced information from the plantar receptors including the intrinsic foot muscles. This evidence suggests that dysfunction or absence of plantar intrinsic muscle activity negatively impacts the control and stabilization of the foot during standing. Plantar information, including information from the plantar intrinsic foot muscles, may play an important role in the absorptive qualities of the muscles outside the foot. This may be caused by the inability of the muscles to contract meaningfully without contextually relevant sensory information about foot deformation.

Intrinsic Foot Muscle Training Enhances Foot Posture

Although alterations of the intrinsic foot muscles through fatigue or paralysis have increased navicular drop during standing, there is evidence to suggest that targeted training of the intrinsic foot muscles has the reverse effect. Mulligan and Cook[19] conducted an intervention study in which healthy subjects underwent progressive intrinsic foot muscle training over the course of 4 weeks and found that navicular drop was significantly reduced after training and continued to decrease over the course of a month after training ceased. Subjects also improved in performance on the postero-medial and posterolateral directions of the Star Excursion Balance Test after the isolated training. Without a control group, it is difficult to determine whether the changes in dynamic balance could be attributed to the training or simply to a learning effect over time. However, based on the results from this study combined with the findings of Fiolkowski and colleagues,[18] there is evidence to support that training the intrinsic foot muscles in healthy individuals can have a reverse effect on foot stability to that of fatiguing the muscles or reducing their function. The continued reduction in navicular drop after training may point to not only beneficial gains in stability, but also gains in sensory information relevant to foot deformation.

Intrinsic Foot Muscle Activation Increases as Postural Demands Increase

The intrinsic foot muscles were originally thought to be not very active during standing and the main supporting structure of the foot during standing is the plantar aponeurosis.[20] However, more recent evidence suggests their activity increases as postural demand increases from sitting, to double-limb standing, to single-limb standing.[21] This suggests that there may be shared load between these degrees of freedom in healthy individuals, which provides redundancy to the strategies available for maintaining arch height while standing. If the plantar intrinsic foot muscles are insufficient or dysfunctional, perhaps the result is increased stress and damage to the plantar aponeurosis and extrinsic foot muscle tendons.

The Timing of Activation and Muscle Cross-Sectional Area Influences Plantar Intrinsic Foot Muscle Function

During walking, the plantar intrinsics demonstrate the highest electromyographic activity during stance phase, especially when the heel lifts off the ground, suggesting that these muscles play a larger role as stabilizers during the propulsion phase of stance rather than the absorption phase.[20,22,23] In those with pes planus, the intrinsic foot muscles activate earlier,[22,23] which suggests that their contributions are greater compared with those with normal feet. New evidence has emerged that although the intrinsic foot muscles contract earlier than those with normal feet, the cross-sectional area of these muscles is considerably smaller.[24] This suggests that these muscles may turn on sooner within the active subsystem of the foot core, but their motor contribution may be compromised in those with pes planus.

Targeted Training Enhances Intrinsic Foot Muscle Cross-Sectional Area

The cross-sectional area of the intrinsic foot muscles can be influenced through intervention. Training the intrinsic foot muscles for 8 weeks in combination with custom-made foot orthotics for those with pes planus increased the cross-sectional area of the abductor hallucis and the flexor hallucis brevis, which are two of the major medial longitudinal arch stabilizers.[25] Importantly, the orthotics alone were also shown to enhance the cross-sectional area of these muscles, but not to the extent of the combination.[25] This evidence suggests supporting the arch via orthotic may afford the body the opportunity to restore the health of the plantar intrinsic muscles; however, the addition of targeted training enhances the capacity of these muscles.[1] It is apparent that the use of foot orthotics for overuse lower extremity conditions is widely accepted in clinical practice with positive outcomes.[12,13] Foot orthotics offer the opportunity for active and passive subsystems of the foot core to recover from increased tissue stress. However, there may not be a corresponding recovery in functional variability within the foot core system with isolated orthotic use.

Electrical Stimulation Enhances the Function of the Intrinsic Foot Muscles as Medial Longitudinal Arch Stabilizers

Electrical stimulation of the intrinsic foot muscles has also been shown to be effective in decreasing longitudinal arch deformation with progressively increased loading of the foot. Kelly and colleagues[26] examined the effects of progressively loading the foot to 1.5 times body weight while subjects were seated. They examined the subsequent changes in foot posture and activity within the abductor hallucis, flexor digitorum brevis, and the quadratus plantae and found that increasing the load on the foot resulted in increased deformation related to hyperpronation of the longitudinal arch and increased electromyographic activity from the three plantar intrinsic muscles.[26] The investigators then stimulated these muscles beyond their natural muscular activity and found that the activation of these muscles led to a greater resistance of foot deformation as the load increased on the foot. These muscles are thought to act as a dynamic truss for the foot, similar to the truss provided by the plantar aponeurosis, but with the ability to actively contract without toe extension or dorsiflexion of the ankle.[26]

TRAINING THE FOOT CORE (FROM ISOLATION TO INTEGRATION)

When planning a rehabilitation program, it is important to address the multifactorial nature of the condition in a systematic and logical way.[27,28] Achieving foundational goals, such as controlling pain, allowing adequate and isolated rest of the damaged tissues, and restoring mobility and control of the affected joints, is paramount.[29] When such factors have been addressed and progressed, isolated volitional muscle training can be introduced with a progression toward functional integration (see **Fig. 6**).[29] We recommend for overuse lower extremity conditions, that foot core training be introduced to promote the restoration of functional variability of foot control.[7,27] When initiating foot core training, an essential element that must be started first is the awareness of the target position for foot control. The target position for foot core training is a neutral foot position between pronation and supination (subtalar neutral).[1,5,30] This is similar to lumbopelvic core stability training in that we train a patient to find pelvic neutral before helping them learn to activate the muscles that maintain that position.[1] Teaching patients how to find subtalar neutral helps them understand what position they are to maintain during exercises.

Finding Subtalar Neutral

To find subtalar neutral, patients while seated and their feet flat on the ground are asked to lift the medial aspect of the plantar surface of the foot off the ground without the lateral (supination) and then the lateral without the medial (pronation) as far as they can without excessive lateral motion at the knee. When they have found the limits, they are then asked to maximally supinate and slowly bring the medial plantar surface of the foot back down to the ground until the ball of the foot slightly touches the ground.[1] This position is typically aligned with subtalar neutral and is also the midpoint between both forefoot and rearfoot supination and pronation. This neutral position is critical to come back to in each repetition of plantar intrinsic muscle training to promote an awareness of the neutral foot position, which is prepared for absorption (pronation) and propulsion (supination).[1]

ISOLATED FOOT CORE TRAINING (THE SHORT FOOT EXERCISE)
Modeling the Foot

In isolated foot core training, the first step is dedicated toward modeling (shaping and controlling) the target position for optimal foot adaptability. An excellent exercise for isolating the plantar intrinsic foot muscles is known as the short (small) foot exercise.[1,5,19,30] In this exercise, volitional control of the plantar intrinsic foot muscles is emphasized to raise the arches of the foot and subsequently shorten the length of the foot. An important initial consideration for training preparation is "awakening" the muscles. Janda and colleagues[30] recommended that mobility of the foot be ensured before initiating any training. Therefore, we recommend combining joint mobilizations of the joints across the foot (gliding the tarsal and metatarsal joints) with large amplitude oscillations to ensure that full motion can be achieved across all joints. Additionally, deep massage of the plantar surface of the foot is also recommended as a way to stimulate the neural subsystem of the foot core system.[30]

Because the short foot exercise is often a difficult concept to grasp, Janda and colleagues[30] recommended three stages of training for these muscles: (1) passive modeling, (2) active-assistive modeling, and (3) active modeling. Passive modeling involves the therapist moving the patient's foot through the short foot motion, shortening and lengthening the foot so that the patient can differentiate between the positions.[30] Active-assistive modeling involves passive modeling from the therapist with active contractions of the plantar intrinsic muscles to actively recreate the short foot position.[30] Active modeling is then achieved when the patient can perform this activity without the assistance of the therapist.[30] Even with these strategies, the short foot contraction can still be difficult to achieve. A novel development in the literature for isolating the plantar intrinsic foot muscles is assisting the contraction of the intrinsic foot muscles with electrical stimulation. In lieu of active-assistive modeling, the muscles are stimulated to contract and produce the short foot position while the patient can then feel and see the change. Gradually, the patient can then be progressed to more volitional control and active modeling in a similar fashion to contracting the quadriceps assisted with neuromuscular electrical stimulation.

Active-Assisted Modeling with Neuromuscular Electrical Stimulation

Neuromuscular electrostimulation (NMES) increases neural activation and strengthens human skeletal muscle.[31,32] It is a promising modality for rehabilitation to strengthen and stimulate the intrinsic medial arch muscles on an involuntary basis.[33–36] It can be used as a compliment to voluntary exercise and further posited as a rehabilitative tool for injuries affecting normal neuromuscular function.[36]

Recent evidence suggests that NMES of foot intrinsic muscles can decrease the navicular drop through a 3-week program including three sessions a week[34] or can be used in combination with other exercises during a 5-week protocol resulting in a lateral shift of the foot plantar pressure patterns. This may support the use of NMES of the intrinsic foot muscle for promoting foot core strength in the long term and subsequently prevent arch collapse and hyperpronation in dynamic conditions. In addition, Gaillet and colleagues[35] reported that a single 20-minute NMES session of the abductor hallucis induced an immediate lateral displacement of anterior maximal pressure point (eg, inversion) in standing position, which persisted "chronically" 2 months later, probably because of the plasticity of spinally mediated abductor hallucis afferent connections. In the same line, a single 20-minute session of high-frequency, low-intensity wide-pulse NMES over the abductor hallucis showed interesting effects on subsequent foot function during walking, such as an increase in forefoot eversion with concomitant rearfoot inversion in the frontal plane and rearfoot-dominated adduction in the transverse plane. These findings confirm the mechanical effect of NMES as an efficient modality in maximizing the sensory volley to the spinal cord eliciting hyperexcitability of abductor hallucis motor units, emphasizing the neurologic-related effect of the NMES rather than the strengthening effect over a single treatment session.[36]

The Neuromuscular Electrostimulation Protocol for Active-Assisted Intrinsic Foot Muscle Training

For NMES active-assisted intrinsic foot muscle training, patients should stand with both feet on the ground. One portable stimulator (eg, Compex 3; Medicompex SA, Ecublens, Switzerland) is used to deliver NEMS (15 minutes; 75 NEMS contractions completed during each training session; rise time = 0.25 seconds and descending time = 0.75 seconds). Two electrodes are placed behind the head of the first metatarsal to stimulate the medial arch intrinsic muscles (**Fig. 2**). To maximize muscle tension without accompanying detrimental effects on fatigue onset, biphasic symmetric regular-wave pulsed currents (85 Hz) lasting 400 μs are delivered.[31,37] Each 4-second steady tetanic stimulation is followed by a rest period lasting 8 seconds, during which subjects are submaximally stimulated at 4 Hz to the medial arch muscles with the foot flat on the ground. The goal for patients is to consistently increase the current amplitude within each training session and between sessions to attain the highest tolerable level of muscle contraction without discomfort. In the rest time between contractions, patients are instructed to repeatedly reestablish subtalar neutral position before the next contraction. They are also encouraged to volitionally contract the intrinsic foot muscles with the NMES to promote the active-assisted modeling to prepare for the transition to active modeling in standing. **Table 1** provides a quick reference for NMES parameters.

Based on our experiences and the current available evidence, patients should perform an average of 9 to 12 NMES sessions throughout 3 to 5 weeks with a gradual progression of active modeling in combination with functional integration activities, such as single-limb squatting. One 20-minute session of NMES produced lasting effects on foot posture and control.[35] Evaluating a patient's ability to volitionally control these muscles at the end of each session is a good way to determine whether NMES should be continued in the next session. Initially, the patients begin in double-limb stance (**Fig. 3**) and progress to more challenging single-limb stance activities. During progression of the treatment, the patient (**Fig. 4**), followed by a single-leg standing position including a flexion of the knee, increased dorsiflexion, and an increased loading on the medial midfoot after a couple of sessions (**Fig. 5**). This progression

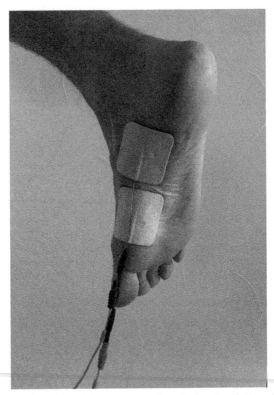

Fig. 2. Placement of electrodes for neuromuscular electrostimulation during the active-assisted modeling phase of isolated training.

targets the recruitment of the medial longitudinal arch muscles in their outer range of motion (ie, arch flattening position caused by the increased percentage of the body mass transferred on the medial midfoot). This "three-position" progression of NMES for active-assisted modeling, ensuring a progressive loading of the medial arch

Table 1
The parameters for neuromuscular electrostimulation of the intrinsic foot muscles during the active-assisted modeling phase of isolated training

Parameters for Neuromuscular Electrostimulation for Active-Assisted Modeling	
Waveform	Symmetric biphasic
Frequency	85 Hz
Pulse length	400 μs
Contraction time	4 s
Ramp up time	0.25 s
Ramp down time	0.75 s
Rest time	8 s
Treatment time	15 min
Contractions	75

The goal of the training is to provide a full tetanic contraction of the intrinsic foot muscles during the contraction time. During the rest period, a 4-Hz submaximal stimulus can be provided.

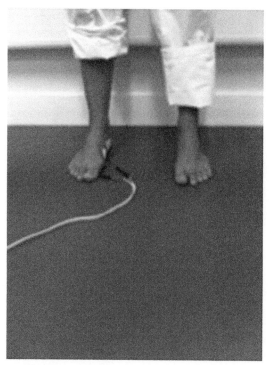

Fig. 3. The double-limb stance position for neuromuscular electrostimulation training during the active-assisted modeling phase of isolated training.

muscles, should then be progressed to entirely voluntary control through a reduction in the NMES over time. Active-assisted NMES training affords a rapid progression from siting to standing on one leg while controlling the intrinsic foot muscles so that the patient can experience what it is like to use these muscles actively.

ACTIVE MODELING AND INTEGRATION TRAINING FOR THE FOOT CORE

As a patient gains volitional control of the plantar intrinsic foot muscles during standing, it is then important to promote the use of these muscles during dynamic activities in which entire foot core system is integrated.[1,29] Although the current protocols for intrinsic foot muscle training generally focus on isolating these muscles during standing, these muscles are also an essential degree of freedom for absorption and propulsion during dynamic activities. One of our observations thus far is that those with poor intrinsic foot muscle control during standing typically also have poor foot posture during a toe raise. During propulsion, the center of pressure under the foot should be directed toward the first metatarsal head when the heel lifts off the ground. However, when examining patients' ability to rise up on their toes, we have often found that those with overuse foot and leg issues often fall out to the lateral metatarsal heads into a more forefoot supinated position. Subsequently, they also adopt more of a wobbly foot posture rather than a stable one. To correct this issue, we place a target under the ball of the foot (a large coin) and ask the patient to raise the heel off the ground and direct the pressure under the foot toward the target. The end result is that patients seem to have a greater ability to distribute the load across the forefoot more medially and adopt a more stable foot posture during propulsion in which

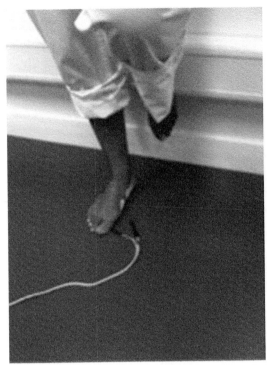

Fig. 4. The single-limb stance position for neuromuscular electrostimulation training during the active-assisted modeling phase of isolated training.

rearfoot supination is combined with forefoot pronation.[36] Training the plantar intrinsic foot muscles with an emphasis on finding subtalar neutral enhances the ability to perform these exercises, which may be the result of adding an additional degree of freedom to the control of the foot during dynamic activities.

As a patient progresses from control of standing for learning to use the intrinsic foot muscles within both the absorption and propulsion phases of stance, it is then essential to transition them to more dynamic activities in which the demands of absorption and propulsion progressively increase. As a patient progresses to more challenging standing activities, it is also important to incorporate control of the intrinsic foot muscles during walking in which the demands of absorption and propulsion are not only increased, but also more rapid in their transitions. From there, progress toward foot core control in such activities as running, hopping, cutting, and landing. To do this, we recommend incorporating a functional hop progression that has been shown to be effective in enhancing functional performance in those with chronic ankle instability.[27,38] In this program, patients are progressed based on their ability to perform hopping and balancing tasks error-free.[38] To promote the control of the foot core, patients are asked to be mindful of their subtalar neutral position and activation of the plantar intrinsic muscles during take-off and landing. During the integration phase of rehabilitation, because there are numerous contributing factors to overuse lower extremity injuries, we recommend that short foot exercises, their isolation, and integration be a component of a multifactorial rehabilitation program that addresses the unique impairments, activity limitations, and participation restrictions of individual patients (**Fig. 6**).

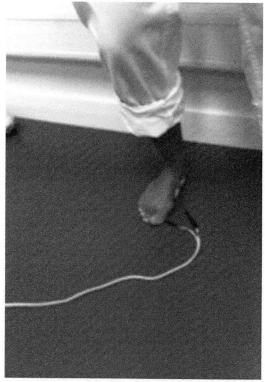

Fig. 5. The single-leg standing position including a flexion of the knee, increased dorsiflexion, and an increased loading on the medial midfoot for neuromuscular electrostimulation training during the active-assisted modeling phase of isolated training.

FUNCTIONAL OUTCOMES FOR FOOT CORE TRAINING

Although we emphasize the importance of isolating and integrating foot core training into rehabilitation for lower extremity overuse injuries (see **Fig. 6**), it is currently unclear which functional outcomes best capture the changes resulting from the intervention in patients. There are numerous techniques for assessing the contributions of the intrinsic foot muscles to the foot core system including strength and foot postural control, but there is limited evidence of these outcomes related to foot core training for patients with overuse or recurrent lower extremity issues. However, the absence of evidence does not necessarily indicate evidence of absence in the benefits that isolating the plantar intrinsic muscles offers for outcomes related to lower extremity overuse conditions.

Using a systematic and logical approach that combines subjective and objective patient outcomes is an excellent way to holistically determine the effectiveness of an intervention. Objective measures, such as navicular drop,[16,19] the foot mobility measure,[39] the intrinsic foot muscle test,[1,5,19,40] the Star Excursion Balance Test,[19,41] and dynamic pedobarography,[42] combined with patient-oriented outcomes, such as symptom perception and self-reported functional ability,[43] would help to establish whether the isolation and integration progression is effective for a patient. For those who seem to respond positively to intrinsic foot muscle training and can integrate those strategies into more complex activities, the effect might be apparent for

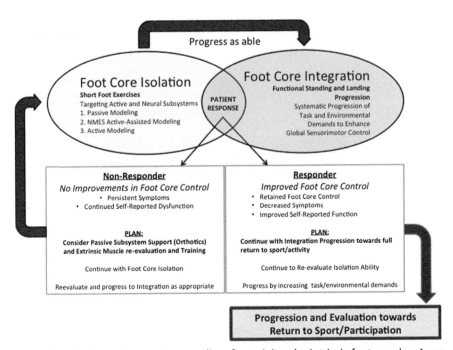

Fig. 6. The isolation to integration paradigm for training the intrinsic foot muscles. As patients progress, it is critically important to evaluate whether they are responding to the isolation training. If they do respond, progress to more advanced isolation and integration activities preparing the patients for return to sport/participation. If the patient does not respond, consider other contributors to foot core stability, such as the passive subsystem and the extrinsic foot muscles and progress as appropriate. It is important to recognize that the foot core system represents the interaction of multiple systems. Training the intrinsic foot muscles provides a means by which their interaction can be enhanced.

the clinician and patient. However, if a patient fails to respond to the isolation to integration progression, it may be that other factors within the foot core system need to be addressed. Perhaps the patient would benefit from a foot orthotic that limits deformation of the foot, improves pain, and reduces strain on active and passive subsystems.[13,44] It may be that there are factors up the chain that need to be isolated and integrated, such as poor lumbopelvic/hip control.[45] The isolation and integration progression has been the hallmark of core stability training.[46] Most importantly, the isolation to integration progression combined with appropriate outcomes affords clinicians the opportunity to evaluate the foot core and choose interventions that are most appropriate for their individual patients.[1]

SUMMARY

Dynamic foot control is critical to the health of the sensorimotor system. Overuse injuries related to foot control may be related to a loss of foot control degrees of freedom, which led to increased tissue stresses on the available structures within the foot core active and passive subsystems. Training the intrinsic foot muscles may offer benefit to the foot core system by increasing the functional variability of degrees of freedom to cope with changing demands of dynamic foot control. Moving from targeted isolation of these muscles to their global integration in movement patterns may offer an excellent strategy for reducing the effects of lower extremity overuse injuries related to poor foot control.

REFERENCES

1. McKeon PO, Hertel J, Bramble D, et al. The foot core system: a new paradigm for understanding intrinsic foot muscle function. Br J Sports Med 2014. [Epub ahead of print]. http://dx.doi.org/10.1136/bjsports-2013-092690.
2. Hicks JH. The mechanics of the foot. I. The joints. J Anat 1953;87(4):345–57.
3. Hicks JH. The mechanics of the foot. II. The plantar aponeurosis and the arch. J Anat 1954;88(1):25–30.
4. Abboud RJ. Relevant foot biomechanics. Curr Orthop 2002;16:165–79.
5. Jam B. Evaluation and retraining of the intrinsic foot muscles for pain syndromes related to abnormal control of pronation. Available at: http://www.aptei.com/articles/pdf/IntrinsicMuscles.pdf. Accessed October 10, 2013.
6. Bolgla LA, Malone TR. Plantar fasciitis and the windlass mechanism: a biomechanical link to clinical practice. J Athl Train 2004;39(1):77–82.
7. Davids K, Glazier P, Araujo D, et al. Movement systems as dynamical systems: the functional role of variability and its implications for sports medicine. Sports Med 2003;33(4):245–60.
8. Davids K, Glazier P. Deconstructing neurobiological coordination: the role of the biomechanics-motor control nexus. Exerc Sport Sci Rev 2010;38(2):86–90.
9. Williams KR. Biomechanics of distance running. In: Grabiner MD, editor. Current issues in biomechanics. 1st edition. Champaign (IL): Human Kinetics; 1993. p. 3–32.
10. Goff JD, Crawford R. Diagnosis and treatment of plantar fasciitis. Am Fam Physician 2011;84(6):676–82.
11. Winters M, Eskes M, Weir A, et al. Treatment of medial tibial stress syndrome: a systematic review. Sports Med 2013;43(12):1315–33.
12. Banwell HA, Mackintosh S, Thewlis D. Foot orthoses for adults with flexible pes planus: a systematic review. J Foot Ankle Res 2014;7(1):23.
13. Collins N, Bisset L, McPoil T, et al. Foot orthoses in lower limb overuse conditions: a systematic review and meta-analysis. Foot Ankle Int 2007;28(3):396–412.
14. McPoil TG, Martin RL, Cornwall MW, et al. Heel pain–plantar fasciitis: clinical practice guildelines linked to the international classification of function, disability, and health from the orthopaedic section of the American Physical Therapy Association. J Orthop Sports Phys Ther 2008;38(4):A1–18.
15. Bowring B, Chockalingam N. A clinical guideline for the conservative management of tibialis posterior tendon dysfunction. Foot (Edinb) 2009;19(4):211–7.
16. Headlee DL, Leonard JL, Hart JM, et al. Fatigue of the plantar intrinsic foot muscles increases navicular drop. J Electromyogr Kinesiol 2008;18(3):420–5.
17. Fiolkowski P, Brunt D, Bishop M, et al. Intrinsic pedal musculature support of the medial longitudinal arch: an electromyography study. J Foot Ankle Surg 2003;42(6):327–33.
18. Fiolkowski P, Bishop M, Brunt D, et al. Plantar feedback contributes to the regulation of leg stiffness. Clin Biomech (Bristol, Avon) 2005;20(9):952–8.
19. Mulligan EP, Cook PG. Effect of plantar intrinsic muscle training on medial longitudinal arch morphology and dynamic function. Man Ther 2013;18(5):425–30.
20. Mann R, Inman VT. Phasic activity of intrinsic muscles of the foot. J Bone Joint Surg Am 1964;46:469–81.

21. Kelly LA, Kuitunen S, Racinais S, et al. Recruitment of the plantar intrinsic foot muscles with increasing postural demand. Clin Biomech (Bristol, Avon) 2012; 27(1):46–51.
22. Basmajian JV, Stecko G. The role of muscles in arch support of the foot. J Bone Joint Surg Am 1963;45:1184–90.
23. Gray EG, Basmajian JV. Electromyography and cinematography of leg and foot ("normal" and flat) during walking. Anat Rec 1968;161(1):1–15.
24. Angin S, Crofts G, Mickle KJ, et al. Ultrasound evaluation of foot muscles and plantar fascia in pes planus. Gait Posture 2014;40(1):48–52.
25. Jung DY, Koh EK, Kwon OY. Effect of foot orthoses and short-foot exercise on the cross-sectional area of the abductor hallucis muscle in subjects with pes planus: a randomized controlled trial. J Back Musculoskelet Rehabil 2011;24(4):225–31.
26. Kelly LA, Cresswell AG, Racinais S, et al. Intrinsic foot muscles have the capacity to control deformation of the longitudinal arch. J R Soc Interf 2014;11(93):20131188.
27. McKeon PO. Dynamic systems theory as a guide to balance training development for chronic ankle instability. Athletic Training and Sports Health Care 2012;4(5):230–6.
28. Wikstrom EA, Hubbard-Turner T, McKeon PO. Understanding and treating lateral ankle sprains and their consequences: a constraints-based approach. Sports Med 2013;43(6):385–93.
29. Hertel J, Denegar CR. A rehabilitation paradigm for restoring neuromuscular control following athletic injury. Athl Ther Today 1998;3(5):12–6.
30. Janda V, Vavrova M, Hervenova A, et al. Sensory motor stimulation. In: Liebenson C, editor. Rehabilitation of the spine: a practitioner's manual. 2nd edition. Baltimore, MD: Lippincott Williams & Wilkins; 2006. p. 517–9.
31. Maffiuletti NA. Physiological and methodological considerations for the use of neuromuscular electrical stimulation. Eur J Appl Physiol 2010;110(2):223–34.
32. Paillard T. Combined application of neuromuscular electrical stimulation and voluntary muscular contractions. Sports Med 2008;38(2):161–77.
33. Fourchet F, Kuitunen S, Girard O, et al. Effects of combined foot/ankle electromyostimulation and resistance training on the in-shoe plantar pressure patterns during sprint in young athletes. J Sports Sci Med 2011;10(2):292–300.
34. Fourchet FK, Loepelt H, Millet GP. Plantar muscles electro-stimulation and navicular drop. Sci Sports 2009;24(5):262–4.
35. Gaillet JC, Biraud JC, Bessou M, et al. Modifications of baropodograms after transcutaneous electric stimulation of the abductor hallucis muscle in humans standing erect. Clin Biomech (Bristol, Avon) 2004;19(10):1066–9.
36. James DC, Chesters T, Sumners DP, et al. Wide-pulse electrical stimulation to an intrinsic foot muscle induces acute functional changes in forefoot-rearfoot coupling behaviour during walking. Int J Sports Med 2013;34(5):438–43.
37. Papaiordanidou M, Guiraud D, Varray A. Kinetics of neuromuscular changes during low-frequency electrical stimulation. Muscle Nerve 2010;41:54–62.
38. McKeon PO, Ingersoll CD, Kerrigan DC, et al. Balance training improves function and postural control in those with chronic ankle instability. Med Sci Sports Exerc 2008;40(10):1810–9.
39. McPoil TG, Vicenzino B, Cornwall MW, et al. Reliability and normative values for the foot mobility magnitude: a composite measure of vertical and medial-lateral mobility of the midfoot. J Foot Ankle Res 2009;2:6.
40. Sauer LD, Beazell J, Hertel J. Considering the intrinsic foot musculature in evaluation and rehabilitation for lower extremity injuries. Athletic Training and Sports Health Care 2011;3(1):43–7.

41. Gribble PA, Hertel J, Plisky P. Using the star excursion balance test to assess dynamic postural-control deficits and outcomes in lower extremity injury: a literature and systematic review. J Athl Train 2012;47(3):339–57.

42. Fourchet F, Kelly L, Horobeanu C, et al. Comparison of plantar pressure distribution in adolescent runners at low vs. high running velocity. Gait Posture 2012; 35(4):685–7.

43. Sauer LD, Saliba SA, Ingersoll CD, et al. Effects of rehabilitation incorporating short foot exercises on self-reported function, static and dynamic balance in chronic ankle instability patients. J Athl Train 2010;45:S67.

44. Lee SY, McKeon P, Hertel J. Does the use of orthoses improve self-reported pain and function measures in patients with plantar fasciitis? A meta-analysis. Phys Ther Sport 2009;10(1):12–8.

45. Willson JD, Dougherty CP, Ireland ML, et al. Core stability and its relationship to lower extremity function and injury. J Am Acad Orthop Surg 2005;13(5):316–25.

46. Kibler WB, Press J, Sciascia A. The role of core stability in athletic function. Sports Med 2006;36(3):189–98.

Treating Tendinopathy
Perspective on Anti-inflammatory Intervention and Therapeutic Exercise

Michael F. Joseph, PhD, PT, Craig R. Denegar, PhD, PT, ATC, FNATA*

KEYWORDS

- Tendinopathy • Anti-inflammatory • Eccentric loading • Therapeutic exercise

KEY POINTS

- Tendinopathy is the clinical term for tendon overuse injuries.
- Histopathologic examination frequently reveals a noninflammatory process underlying tendinosis; however, an inflammatory infiltrate has been demonstrated in pathologic supraspinatus, subscapularis, and Achilles tendons.
- There is a poor relationship between symptoms and the onset of tendon pathology; however, a continuum from early reactive tendinopathy to late degenerative tendinosis may be identified with clinical examination and imaging.
- Anti-inflammatory medication may have a role in the early stages of tendinosis; however, several deleterious effects have been noted, including increased risk of rupture, adipogenisis, and chondrogenesis.
- Mechanical loading through exercises inclusive of eccentrics and heavy slow resistance are efficacious in the treatment of Achilles and patellar tendinopathy.

INTRODUCTION AND TERMINOLOGY

The tendon transmits force developed through muscle contraction to bone, resulting in motion and joint stabilization. Tendon is inherently exposed to large magnitude loads and has the ability to adapt in form and behavior in response to loading history. The mechanism of tendon adaptation is largely through autocrine/paracrine signaling via mechanotransduction pathways.[1] Excessive or insufficient loading disrupts tissue homeostasis and is a primary factor in the development of tendon pathology. Diseased tendon is typified by cellular dysfunction and tissue alterations, leading to functional compromise. It is alarming that most tendon ruptures occur without warning symptoms, yet postrupture tendon shows signs of chronic degeneration.[2]

Department of Kinesiology, University of Connecticut, 2095 Hillside Road, U-1110, Storrs, CT 06269-1110, USA
* Corresponding author.
E-mail address: craig.denegar@uconn.edu

Clin Sports Med 34 (2015) 363–374
http://dx.doi.org/10.1016/j.csm.2014.12.006
0278-5919/15/$ – see front matter © 2015 Elsevier Inc. All rights reserved.

Tendinosis is a degenerative condition with a notable absence of inflammatory cells and what has been characterized as a failed healing response.[3,4] Several studies have documented the absence of an inflammatory response in human ruptured tendons,[2,5] biopsy samples,[6] or surgical debridement samples.[7,8] A paradigm shift away from an inflammatory model of tendinitis has occurred and the treatment of tendon related symptoms reassessed in light of new understanding. Because the diagnosis of tendinosis requires histopathologic examination, the term tendinopathy is advocated for the clinical presentation of tendon pain, stiffness, and loss of function related to mechanical loading.[9]

A combination of intrinsic and extrinsic factors lead to the development of tendinopathy. Influential intrinsic factors favoring the development of tendinopathy as well as tendon rupture include advancing age and gender. Men are significantly more prone to both tendinopathy and rupture. Additionally, genetics (variations in genes for tissue and cellular proteins) and limb mechanics affect risk. Extrinsic factors such as activity level, footwear, training technique, and surface type have been implicated in both Achilles and patella tendinopathy. Loading history is likely a key component in the pathogenesis of tendinopathy, with a likely interaction with intrinsic factors.

The tendon adapts to mechanical load through alterations in composition and mechanical properties. There seems to be a threshold to overuse, and the quantification of appropriate load (volume, intensity, and frequency) for optimal tendon function remains elusive. Appropriate load is anabolic. Overloading has catabolic effects on the tendon tissue, as degradation of the extracellular matrix exceeds synthesis of new tissue. Seemingly contradictory is the benefit seen with eccentric exercise. At first glance, adding load to an overloaded tissue is counterintuitive. In a degenerative condition in which cell and tissue interactions are disrupted, stimulation of the tendon cell (tenocyte) through eccentric loading is likely anabolic and therefore advantageous. Achilles and patella tendinopathy are prevalent in an athletic population and respond well to loading programs.[5]

The purpose of this article is to review the pathogenesis of tendinopathy and discuss the possibility that inflammatory mediators are at work despite the absence of leukocytes in tissue samples. We review the role of anti-inflammatory medications in the management of tendinopathy and then describe effective loading programs for the management of Achilles and patella tendinopathy.

TENDINOSIS

Although viewed as a local lesion, tendinosis affects the entire tendon. Macroscopically, tendon darkens and loses its pearly white appearance.[10,11] The peritendinous and intratendinous tissue may be affected in isolation or concomitantly. The peritendinous tissue thickens and can cause adhesions, which may constrict the microvasculature.[10] A proliferation of fibroblasts and myofibroblasts in the paratenon is thought to be responsible.

Proliferation of neovascularity is often present, and some feel this vascular proliferation may be the pain generator of tendinopathic tendon.[12] It is important to note that a large percentage of tendinosis is asymptomatic, and 90% of spontaneous tendon ruptures can occur prior to any precipitating symptomatology. Underlying degenerative tissue is typically found.[2]

In a diseased tendon, collagen becomes disorganized, with visible microtearing, decreased density and fiber diameter, and loss of crimp. An increase in reparative type 3 collagen is noted. The alterations in organization and composition of collagen compromise tendon structural integrity.[13] Several variations of collagen degeneration have been described (hypoxic, mucoid, myxoid, hyaline, lipoid fibrocartilagenous, and calcific).[10] These varying forms of degeneration may coexist depending upon anatomic location and etiopathogenesis.

Altered loading in tendinotic tendon leads to the increased production of several large modular proteoglycans (PGs) such as aggrecan.[10,14,15] The prolific increase in PGs is often associated with fibrocartilaginous metaplasia or in streaming bands throughout the tendon midsubstance. Pooling of PG contributes to collagen disorganization and impaired structural integrity.

Variable cellular changes have been reported inclusive of hypercellularity, hypocellularity, apoptosis, and necrosis.[16] The tenocyte may become rounded or chondroid in appearance and contain pronounced endoplasmic reticulum consistent with hyperproduction of proteoglycan.

A more complete understanding of the pathogenesis of tendon is hampered by its often asymptomatic nature and the practicality of obtaining human tendon for analysis. Tendinopathic tissue is often obtained after rupture and therefore represents end-stage pathology. Postrupture tissue differs in protein expression compared with painful nonruptured tendon.[17] The end-stage histologic picture of tendinosis is likely not indicative of the precipitating pathologic process, as evidenced by the multiple forms of tissue degeneration that have been noted. The changes in cellular content and extracellular matrix alter the mechanical properties of tendon. The tendon becomes less stiff and less efficient in force transfer.

TENDINOPATHY—A CONTINUUM MODEL

Recently, a continuum model of tendinopathy has been proposed[18] and has gained support.[19] The proposed continuum of pathology is described in 3 stages, which are likely overlapping: reactive tendinopathy, tendon disrepair (failed healing), and degenerative tendinopathy. Degenerative tendinopathy represents tendinosis. The modulation of load is the primary driver moving tendon forward or backward along the continuum.

Reactive tendinopathy is proposed to occur in response to acute overload and is described as a noninflammatory proliferative response. In vitro work supports this observation of hypercellularity, absence of inflammatory infiltrate, and the shift toward synthesis of large modular PGs.

Tendon disrepair or failed healing is the second stage of the continuum proposed by Cook and Purdam,[18] which resembles the initial stage of reactivity but with greater matrix disorganization. Neovascularity and neuronal ingrowth occur and represent an aspect of attempted but failed repair.[5] Evidence exists that the tendon can recover in form and function from this stage with appropriate treatment inclusive of load modulation and eccentric exercise stimulus.

Degenerative tendinopathy (tendinosis) is the final stage in this continuum. Features include vast areas of hypocellularity,[20] pooling of proteglycan, and severely disorganized collagen.[10] It is thought these changes are largely irreversible.

From a clinical perspective, this model divides tendinopathy in 2 distinct groups, early reactive, and late disrepair/degeneration. Local swelling and mildly focal hypoechoic lesions on ultrasound in a younger individual indicate early reactive tendinopathy. A thick nodular tendon with large defined areas of hypoechogenicity and evidence of vascular ingrowth typically identified in older individuals represents late degenerative tendinopathy. In either clinical picture, symptoms can be variable and occur at any point in the continuum.

The acute reactive and late degenerative phases may require different treatment approaches. Although chronic degenerative tendinopathy responds to treatment modalities geared toward stimulating the tissue and cells (eg, eccentric exercise or extracorporeal shockwave therapy [ESWT]), acute reactive tendinopathy that involves a proliferative response of tissue and cellular components may worsen with repetitive mechanical stimulation.[21] Additionally, early reactive tendinopathy may respond favorably to nonsteroidal anti-inflammatory drugs (NSAIDs), which is counterintuitive based upon the noninflammatory nature of the pathology. NSAIDs retard healing in a number of soft tissues[22] but may be advantageous early on in stemming the overproliferation of PGs and ground substance associated with this phase of the pathology.[18]

As discussed, challenges in managing tendinopathy center around difficulties in determining the acuity of the process, and therefore treatments are prescribed independent of a clear delineation in pathophysiology. Although current opinion based upon considerable evidence supports a degenerative process throughout, the presence of an inflammatory process in the early reactive period cannot be ruled out. Practically, a young athlete presenting with an acute onset of local tendon swelling and perhaps pain may benefit in the short term from decreasing repetitive tendon stress. This can be accomplished by decreasing the intensity of exercise and increasing rest periods between activities that load the affected tissues until symptoms resolve.

Recent studies using flow cytometry and immunohistochemical staining of human tendon samples have provided new perspectives of tendinopathy. Findings from recent studies of human Achilles and supraspinatus tears challenge a strictly noninflammatory model of tendon pathology. Inflammatory cells have been observed in torn supraspinatus and postruptured and chronic nonruptured Achilles tendinopathy.[23,24] In a sample of 60 consecutive Achilles tendon ruptures, immunohistochemical staining confirmed the presence of neutrophils, macrophages, and T and B lymphocytes.[23] Biopsy samples from small rotator cuff tears show a considerable inflammatory infiltrate of macrophages and mast cells compared with large tears, which are more degenerated.[25] Regardless of the presence or absence of inflammatory cells, there remains an insufficient stimulation for repair.

Millar and colleagues[26] showed inflammatory cell infiltrate in torn supraspinatus that was inversely proportional to the size of the tear. Additionally, adjacent subscapularis tissue had a greater inflammatory cell count compared with healthy control tendon obtained from the subscapularis of individuals having shoulder stabilization procedures without cuff tear. Torn supraspinatus and adjacent subscapularis tissue had an increased expression of several inflammatory cytokines and apoptotic genes.[27] Tumor necrosis factor (TNF)-alpha was found in subscapularis, not supraspinatus, and is linked to early inflammatory activity. Despite normal appearance on MRI and arthroscopy, adjacent subscapularis tissue exhibited advanced degenerative changes. Subscapularis samples from surgical procedures not involving the rotator cuff were free of degenerative changes or inflammatory cell proliferation.

The presence of proinflammatory agents in the peritendinous tissues has been documented. In tendons from patients with patellar tendinopathy, higher levels of COX-2 and PGE2 expression were seen in the tendon tissue and harvested cells.[28] High levels of the excitatory neurotransmitter glutamate and its receptor are in tendons from patients with Achilles tendinopathy.[29] Neuropeptides have been found to exert proinflammatory actions in addition to their nociceptive functions.[30,31]

ANTI-INFLAMMATORY INTERVENTIONS
Corticosteroids

Although predominantly recognized as a degenerative, rather than a principally inflammatory condition, there is some evidence of pain relief following corticosteroid injection in patients suffering from rotator cuff,[32,33] elbow,[32] Achilles tendinopathy,[34,35] and patella tendinopathy. The mechanism of action is unclear. If inflammatory cytokines are present, then one would expect pain relief in response to corticosteroid administration. Skjong and colleagues[36] suggested that an inflammatory response in tissues surrounding the degenerative tendon tissue may be responsible for the pain associated with the condition. The suppression of inflammation through intratendinous or peritendinous injection would explain the analgesic response to corticosteroid injection. The effects appear more pronounced in the short term (ie, 1–12 weeks) compared with the long term (>12 weeks) but were associated with impaired long-term collagen synthesis and cross-linking, leading to structural weakness.

The protracted report of symptoms and functional loss reported by patients suffering from tendinopathy has led to continued interest in injectable remedies. It is recognized, however, that corticosteroid interferes with tissue repair, and the injection of these medications is associated with an increased risk of tendon rupture. Clinical trials involving corticosteroid injection for the treatment of shoulder and Achilles tendinopathy lack sufficient follow-up and sample size to clearly define the magnitude of risk elevation. This is important, as it has been recognized that most tendons that go on to rupture in adults demonstrate prefailure degenerative changes.[37] The mechanism through which corticosteroids shift risk of rupture has not been fully elucidated, but Zhang and colleagues[38] demonstrated a shift away from gene expression associated with type 1 collagen synthesis toward expression associated with adipogenisis and chondrogenisis in patella tendon progenitor cells exposed to dexamethasone. The magnitude of effect was dose-dependent, with greater exposure associated with more deleterious responses.

The progressive degeneration toward rupture is likely complex, but the long-term risks associated with corticosteroid injection must considered in the light of potential short-term pain relief and the potential of other interventions to affect symptom resolution without increasing risk of reinjury or rupture.

Phoresis

Iontophoresis (the use of direct current) and phonophoresis (the use of an acoustic wave) have been used in conjunction with corticosteroid medications in the treatment of tendinopathy. These modalities seek to drive medication through the dermis to the affected tissue. Dexamethasone possesses a negative electrical charge in solution and is most commonly used for iontophoresis, while hydrocortisone, dexamethasone, and other topical steroidal preparations have been used with phonophoresis.

Similar to investigations into corticosteroid injection in the treatment of tendinopathy, the clinical research related to iontophoresis is conflicting.[39] The methodological quality of many studies, as well as the previously mentioned effect of dexamethasone in tendon progenitor cell activity, is concerning. Beyond these concerns, however, is the fact that the delivery of a pharmacologically active dose of medication to tendon tissue has not been demonstrated. Although the effect of iontophoresis and phonophoresis treatments on the risk of tendon rupture has not been reported, the widespread use of these interventions has not led to the same concerns associated with corticosteroid injection. The most plausible explanation for this observation is that iontophoresis and phonophoresis have a better safety profile, because these treatments are ineffective in delivering medication to the damaged tendon. Thus iontophoresis and phonophoresis with corticosteroids cannot be recommended based upon

A lack of clear benefit demonstrated through clinical research
Concerns related to the impact of corticosteroids on tendon progenitor cell function
Lack of drug delivery data to establish dose response

Nonsteroidal Anti-inflammatory Medications

Oral and topical administration may provide short-term pain relief for patients suffering from tendinopathy,[36,40] although not all investigators report a positive effect.[41] The mechanism is unclear, although the notion of inflammation in surrounding tissue offers a possible explanation. It has also been suggested that non-steroidal anti-inflammatory drugs (NSAIDs) suppress an inflammatory response when tendenopathic tissue is loaded through exercise. Pingel and colleagues[42] found that inflammatory signaling was blunted in tendinopathic versus healthy tendon following exercise and unaffected by 1 week of NSAID administration prior to running.

In addition to the controversies related to true treatment effectiveness and mechanism of action of NSAIDs in patients with tendinopathy, the potential for impaired healing has been explored. Animal models reveal impaired healing related to NSAID administration.[43–45] Zhang and colleagues[46] found that celecoxib impairs tendon-derived stem cell differentiation but did not affect cell proliferation. Interestingly Chechik and colleagues[44] and Connizzo and colleagues[45] suggested that timing of drug administration mediated the deleterious effects of NSAID administration, with Connizzo and colleagues[45] reporting that earlier administration had a greater impact on repair, while Chechik and colleagues[44] reported greater effects when NSAIDs are administered 11 to 20 days (as opposed to 0–10 days) after surgery.

Summary: Anti-inflammatory Interventions

It is apparent that steroidal and nonsteroidal medications can have short-term analgesic effects in some patients with tendinopathy, although the extent of response varies. These drugs have less impact as follow-up is temporally extended. The mechanism of effect is uncertain but likely tied to the view that tendinopathy is progressive, degenerative, characterized by a continuum of early inflammatory cytokine presence, and followed by a failure to repair. It is apparent that these drugs can impair healing, although the extent of effect is medication-, dose-, and perhaps timing-specific. The mechanisms by which healing is impaired have not been fully elucidated. Increasingly, attention has shifted to understanding the impact on tendon stem cells and gene expression. The decision to administer, or not administer anti-inflammatory medications is a clinical judgment balancing the need for short-term symptom management and potential long-term consequences.

LOADING PROGRAMS FOR ACHILLES AND PATELLAR TENDINOPATHY

Healthy human tendon increases both inflammatory markers and collagen turnover in response to loading. Load-induced inflammatory activity regulates blood flow during increased functional demand. Inflammatory-mediated increases in collagen turnover are beneficial to remodeling. The removal of the inflammatory response to physiologic tissue loading may be detrimental for this collagen response. Collagen turnover in the core tendon tissue is markedly lower, and inflammatory pathways are likely negligible.[47] Unlike healthy tendon, overloaded tendinopathic tendon does not display enhanced inflammatory activity at rest or after activity. Likely an acute inflammatory condition would not respond to increased loading.

The Achilles and patellar tendons are responsive to loading programs. The predominant form of conservative treatment for tendinopathy has been eccentric loading; however, the mechanism for benefit is unclear. Much of the evidence for the effectiveness of eccentric exercises programs in the treatment of Achilles and patella tendinopathy comes from the works of Alfredson and colleagues.[5,48]

ACHILLES TENDON LOADING

The Achilles tendon is the most commonly affected lower extremity structure. The Achilles tendon attaches the gastrocnemius and soleus muscles to the calcaneus. The Achilles is the largest and strongest tendon in the human body. Achilles tendinopathy encompasses peritendinitis and tendinosis and is the most commonly diagnosed Achilles disorder (55%–65%), followed by insertional pathology (retrocalcaneal bursitis, bone spurs, and insertional tendinopathy, 25%).[10]

The magnitude of loading experienced by the Achilles tendon during activity likely plays a role in the etiopathogenesis of its degeneration and tendinopathy. Direct in vivo force measurements demonstrate loading during running up to 9 kilonewtons [KN] (12.5× body weight [BW]) with 11.1 KN/cm^2 of stress.[49] Repetitive hopping, squat jumping and counter-movement jumps yield 3.79, 2.2, and 1.9 KN respectively.[50]

Tendinopathy is prevalent in both athletic and sedentary populations, with a cumulative lifetime incidence of 5.9%,[51] and a prevalence of 30% in a nonactive population and 50% in elite endurance athletes.[52] An annual incidence of Achilles tendinopathy of between 7% and 9% in top level runners,[53,54] and a lifetime incidence of 40% in elite gymnasts have been reported.[55] Achilles pathology occurs more frequently in men. Between 68% and 79% of Achilles ruptures occur in men.[56,57] Asymptomatic Achilles tendon pathology is more than twice as likely to occur in men,[58] which may explain the large discrepancy in rupture rates.

Eccentric loading of the Achilles tendon is accomplished through heel drops. Heel drops are performed unilaterally off of a step or a box or with a calf raise machine if available. Heel drops are performed with the knee straight to target the gastrocnemius component, and with the knee bent to target the soleus contribution to the Achilles tendon. The contralateral limb, rather than a concentric contraction, is used to return to the starting position. Frequently prescribed exercise parameters proven successful are 3 sets of 15 repetitions, knee straight and knee bent, twice daily. Stevens and Tan[59] suggested that completing 2 sessions of the exercises daily as tolerated resulted in similar improvements at 6 weeks when compared with patients completing all 180 repetitions daily. Regardless of the protocol, the frequency of eccentric exercise targeting the tendon is much different than utilized for muscle, as with the tendon, the goal is to provide a frequent dose of mechanical stimulus to the tendon cell. External resistance as tolerated may be added by use of a weighted backpack if a calf raise machine is not available.

Along with external resistance, progressive loading is achieved through the rate of eccentric contraction. Based upon force velocity characteristics, increases in force accompany increased speed of contraction. Pain or discomfort is allowed during the activity, but pain persisting after heel drops indicates a slower progression is needed. This may be accomplished through decreasing external resistance, the speed of the exercise, or both.

An alternative loading regime to the classic Alfredson[48] heel drop program was proposed by Silbernagel.[59] This program has 3 phases. The initial phase is similar to a warm up, designed to increase blood flow, ankle range of motion (ROM), and tissue compliance. Included are active range of motion (AROM) of toe extension/flexion and ankle dorsi and plantarflexion; 3 sets 20 seconds of gastrocnemius and soleus stretching, single leg balance, heel and toe walking, and concentric/eccentric heel raises all performed 3 times per day.

Phase 2 includes all exercises in phase 1 with a progression to unilateral eccentric toe raises. Phase 2 lasts 2 weeks. Phase 3, from weeks 4 to 12 continues to progress the toe raise exercises and introduces a plyometric component of quick rebounding toe raises, 20 to 100 repetitions performed 3 times per day. Patients are instructed that pain up to 5/10 on a visual analog scale during and after exercise is acceptable. Patients are further advised that increases in pain and stiffness on the day following exercise indicates that the exercise regimen exceeded tissue tolerance, and exercise volume and intensity should be reduced by returning to an earlier phase of the program.

A recent systematic review[60] compared loading programs and concluded that

Greater satisfaction and return to function occurs with eccentric compared with concentric exercise

Greater patient satisfaction and visual analog scale (VAS) pain outcomes occur with the Silbernagel[59] combined loading program compared with concentric/eccentric calf raises and stretching

Greater reductions in VAS pain scores and faster return to play occur with eccentric/concentric loading compared with isotonic loading

PATELLA TENDON LOADING

The patellar tendon is the continuation of the quadriceps tendon attaching to the patella and tibial tubercle. Because of bony proximal and distal insertions, some consider the patella tendon to be a ligament. Tendinopathy occurs most frequently at the bony insertions, proximally at the attachment to the inferior patellar pole and distally at the tuberosity. Patella tendinopathy affects 12% of elite athletes among an assortment of sports, and as many as 40% of elite athletes in jumping sports such as basketball and volleyball.[61,62] The prevalence in recreational athletes in 1 study was 8.5%.[63]

Success has been demonstrated with both eccentric decline squats and heavy slow resistance training (HSRT) for patella tendinopathy.[64] Parameters for decline squats are similar to those described for the Achilles tendon: 3 sets of 15 repetitions, twice daily. Squats are performed on an incline board to preferentially load the quadriceps. HSRT mimics a more traditional strength training routine. Squats, hack squats, and leg presses are performed 3 times per week. Both eccentric and concentric contractions occur over 3 seconds. Four sets of each exercise with increasing loads are progressed across 12 weeks. Exercise progresses as following

Week 1, 15-repetition maximum (RM)
Weeks 2 to 3, 12 RM
Weeks 4 to 5, 10 RM
Weeks 6 to 8, 8 RM
Weeks 9 to 12, 6 RM

RM is described as the maximum weight that can be used to complete the prescribed number of repetitions. For example, if a patient can leg press 180 pounds 15 times but fails in attempting the 16th repetition, the RM = 180 pounds. As patients progress, the RM will increase if the number of repetitions is held constant. Progression of the protocol leads to using greater resistance for fewer repetitions. There is moderate evidence to support heavy slow resistance training (HSRT) over eccentric exercise alone.[65]

Although most loading protocols allow tendon pain or discomfort during the activity, pain persisting after loading indicates a slower progression is warranted. Care must be taken to choose exercises that not only load the tendon appropriately, but take into account the stress imposed on surrounding tissue and adjacent joints. For example, heavy loading of the patella tendon may easily irritate the patellofemoral joint and surrounding soft tissue. Provoking patellofemoral pain while treating patella tendinopathy is thus counterproductive.

SUMMARY

Evidence of chronic degeneration in the tendon should not imply that early inflammation does not occur. The asymptomatic nature of tendinopathy makes identification of a sentinel inflammatory injury difficult. Torn and adjacent tendon exhibits inflammatory cell infiltrate, more robustly along the periphery of the tendon. Proinflammatory mediators are present within the tendon and peritendon. Healthy tendon behaves differently with respect to these proinflammatory mediators. Whereas healthy tendon responds to loading through enhanced inflammatory activity, tendinopathic tendon does not. Regardless of the possible presence of inflammation in acute stages of tendinopathy, an impaired inflammatory response likely leads to the degenerative condition often seen clinically. Factors that make critical appraisal difficult are human versus animal studies, in vitro versus in vivo systems, variable loading protocols, and anatomic location both within and among tendons.

REFERENCES

1. Wang JH. Mechanobiology of tendon. J Biomech 2006;39:1563–82.
2. Jozsa L, Kannus P. Histopathological findings in spontaneous tendon ruptures. Scand J Med Sci Sports 1997;7:113–8.
3. Hashimoto T, Nobuhara K, Hamada T. Pathologic evidence of degeneration as a primary cause of rotator cuff tear. Clin Orthop Relat Res 2003;(415):111–20.
4. Maffulli N, Wong J, Almekinders LC. Types and epidemiology of tendinopathy. Clin Sports Med 2003;22:675–92.
5. Alfredson H. The chronic painful Achilles and patellar tendon: research on basic biology and treatment. Scand J Med Sci Sports 2005;15:252–9.
6. Martinoli C, Derchi LE, Pastorino C, et al. Analysis of echotexture of tendons with US. Radiology 1993;186:839–43.
7. Benazzo F, Stennardo G, Valli M. Achilles and patellar tendinopathies in athletes: pathogenesis and surgical treatment. Bull Hosp Jt Dis 1996;54:236–40.
8. Cook JL, Khan KM, Harcourt P, et al. A cross sectional study of 100 athletes with jumper's knee managed conservatively and surgically. The Victorian Institute of Sport Tendon Study Group. Br J Sports Med 1997;31:332–6.
9. Maffulli N, Khan KM, Puddu G. Overuse tendon conditions: time to change a confusing terminology. Arthroscopy 1998;14:840–3.
10. Järvinen M, Jozsa L, Kannus P, et al. Histopathological findings in chronic tendon disorders. Scand J Med Sci Sports 1997;7:86–95.
11. Khan KM, Bonar F, Desmond PM, et al. Patellar tendinosis (jumper's knee): findings at histopathologic examination, US, and MR imaging. Victorian Institute of Sport Tendon Study Group. Radiology 1996;200:821–7.
12. Alfredson H, Ohberg L. Sclerosing injections to areas of neo-vascularisation reduce pain in chronic Achilles tendinopathy: a double-blind randomised controlled trial. Knee Surg Sports Traumatol Arthrosc 2005;13:338–44.
13. Sharma P, Maffulli N. Biology of tendon injury: healing, modeling and remodeling. J Musculoskelet Neuronal Interact 2006;6:181–90.
14. Berenson MC, Blevins FT, Plaas AH, et al. Proteoglycans of human rotator cuff tendons. J Orthop Res 1996;14:518–25.
15. Fallon J, Blevins FT, Vogel K, et al. Functional morphology of the supraspinatus tendon. J Orthop Res 2002;20(5):920–6.

16. Galliani I, Burattini S, Mariani AR, et al. Morpho-functional changes in human tendon tissue. Eur J Histochem 2002;46:3–12.
17. Jones GC, Corps AN, Pennington CJ, et al. Expression profiling of metalloproteinases and tissue inhibitors of metalloproteinases in normal and degenerate human achilles tendon. Arthritis Rheum 2006;54(3):832–42.
18. Cook JL, Purdam CR. Is tendon pathology a continuum? A pathology model to explain the clinical presentation of load-induced tendinopathy. Br J Sports Med 2009;43:409–16.
19. McCreesh K, Lewis J. Continuum model of tendon pathology—where are we now? Int J Exp Pathol 2013;94:242–7.
20. Lian O, Scott A, Engebretsen L, et al. Excessive apoptosis in patellar tendinopathy in athletes. Am J Sports Med 2007;35:605–11.
21. Fredberg U, Bolvig L, Andersen NT. Prophylactic training in asymptomatic soccer players with ultrasonographic abnormalities in Achilles and patellar tendons: the Danish Super League Study. Am J Sports Med 2008;36:451–60.
22. Ferry ST, Dahners LE, Afshari HM, et al. The effects of common anti-inflammatory drugs on the healing rat patellar tendon. Am J Sports Med 2007;35:1326–33.
23. Cetti R, Junge J, Vyberg M. Spontaneous rupture of the Achilles tendon is preceded by widespread and bilateral tendon damage and ipsilateral inflammation: a clinical and histopathologic study of 60 patients. Acta Orthop Scand 2003;74:78–84.
24. Schubert TE, Weidler C, Lerch K, et al. Achilles tendinosis is associated with sprouting of substance P positive nerve fibres. Ann Rheum Dis 2005;64:1083–6.
25. Matthews TJ, Hand GC, Rees JL, et al. Pathology of the torn rotator cuff tendon: reduction in potential for repair as tear size increases. J Bone Joint Surg Br 2006;88:489–95.
26. Millar NL, Hueber AJ, Reilly JH, et al. Inflammation is present in early human tendinopathy. Am J Sports Med 2010;38:2085–91.
27. Millar NL, Wei AQ, Molloy TJ, et al. Cytokines and apoptosis in supraspinatus tendinopathy. J Bone Joint Surg Br 2009;91:417–24.
28. Fu SC, Wang W, Pau HM, et al. Increased expression of transforming growth factor-beta1 in patellar tendinosis. Clin Orthop Relat Res 2002;(400):174–83.
29. Alfredson H, Lorentzon R. Chronic tendon pain: no signs of chemical inflammation but high concentrations of the neurotransmitter glutamate. Implications for treatment? Curr Drug Targets 2002;3:43–54.
30. Strand FL, Rose KJ, Zuccarelli LA, et al. Neuropeptide hormones as neurotrophic factors. Physiol Rev 1991;71:1017–46.
31. Schwartz JP. Neurotransmitters as neurotrophic factors: a new set of functions. Int Rev Neurobiol 1992;34:1–23.
32. Gaujoux-Viala C, Dougados M, Gossec L. Efficacy and safety of steroid injections for shoulder and elbow tendonitis: a meta-analysis of randomised controlled trials. Ann Rheum Dis 2009;68:1843–9.
33. Arroll B, Goodyear-Smith F. Corticosteroid injections for painful shoulder: a meta-analysis. Br J Gen Pract 2005;55:224–8.
34. Metcalfe D, Achten J, Costa ML. Glucocorticoid injections in lesions of the Achilles tendon. Foot Ankle Int 2009;30:661–5.
35. Read MT, Motto SG. Tendo Achillis pain: steroids and outcome. Br J Sports Med 1992;26:15–21.
36. Skjong CC, Meininger AK, Ho SS. Tendinopathy treatment: where is the evidence? Clin Sports Med 2012;31:329–50.

37. Kannus P, Józsa L. Histopathological changes preceding spontaneous rupture of a tendon. A controlled study of 891 patients. J Bone Joint Surg Am 1991;73: 1507–25.
38. Zhang J, Keenan C, Wang JH. The effects of dexamethasone on human patellar tendon stem cells: implications for dexamethasone treatment of tendon injury. J Orthop Res 2013;31:105–10.
39. Andres BM, Murrell GA. Treatment of tendinopathy: what works, what does not, and what is on the horizon. Clin Orthop Relat Res 2008;466:1539–54.
40. Maquirriain J, Kolalj A. Management of acute Achilles tendinopathy: effect of etoricoxib on pain control and leg stiffness. Georgian Med News 2013;(222):36–43.
41. Astrom M, Westlin N. No effect of piroxicam on achilles tendinopathy. A randomized study of 70 patients. Acta Orthop Scand 1992;63:631–4.
42. Pingel J, Fredberg U, Mikkelsen LR, et al. No inflammatory gene-expression response to acute exercise in human Achilles tendinopathy. Eur J Appl Physiol 2013;113:2101–9.
43. Dimmen S, Engebretsen L, Nordsletten L, et al. Negative effects of parecoxib and indomethacin on tendon healing: an experimental study in rats. Knee Surg Sports Traumatol Arthrosc 2009;17:835–9.
44. Chechik O, Dolkart O, Mozes G, et al. Timing matters: NSAIDs interfere with the late proliferation stage of a repaired rotator cuff tendon healing in rats. Arch Orthop Trauma Surg 2014;134:515–20.
45. Connizzo BK, Yannascoli SM, Tucker JJ, et al. The detrimental effects of systemic Ibuprofen delivery on tendon healing are time-dependent. Clin Orthop Relat Res 2014;472:2433–9.
46. Zhang K, Zhang S, Li Q, et al. Effects of celecoxib on proliferation and tenocytic differentiation of tendon-derived stem cells. Biochem Biophys Res Commun 2014;450:762–6.
47. Kjaer M, Bayer ML, Eliasson P, et al. What is the impact f inflammation on the critical interplay between mechanical signaling and biochemical changes in tendon matrix? J Appl Physiol 2013;115:879–83.
48. Alfredson H, Pietila T, Jonsson P, et al. Heavy-load eccentric calf muscle training for the treatment of chronic Achilles tendinosis. Am J Sports Med 1998;26:360–6.
49. Komi PV, Fukashiro S, Jarvinen M. Biomechanical loading of Achilles tendon during normal locomotion. Clin Sports Med 1992;11:521–31.
50. Fukashiro S, Komi PV, Jarvinen, et al. In vivo Achilles tendon loading during jumping in humans. Eur J Appl Physiol Occup Physiol 1995;71:453–8.
51. Kujala UM, Sarna S, Kaprio J. Cumulative incidence of Achilles tendon rupture and tendinopathy in male former elite athletes. Clin J Sport Med 2005;15:133–5.
52. Tan SC, Chan O. Achilles and patellar tendinopathy: current understanding of pathophysiology and management. Disabil Rehabil 2008;30:1608–15.
53. Johansson C. Injuries in elite orienteers. Am J Sports Med 1986;14:410–5.
54. Lysholm J, Wiklander J. Injuries in runners. Am J Sports Med 1987;15:168–71.
55. Emerson C, Morrissey D, Perry M, et al. Ultrasonographically detected changes in Achilles tendons and self-reported symptoms in elite gymnasts compared with controls—an observational study. Man Ther 2010;15:37–42.
56. Nyyssonen T, Luthje P, Kroger H. The increasing incidence and difference in sex distribution of Achilles tendon rupture in Findland in 1987-1999. Scand J Surg 2008;97:272–5.
57. Clayton R, Court-Brown C. The epidemiology of musculoskeletal tendinous and ligamentous injuries. Injury 2008;39:1338–44.

58. Gaida JE, Alfredson H, Kiss ZS, et al. Asymptomatic Achilles tendon pathology is associated with a central fat distribution in men and a peripheral fat distribution in women: a cross sectional study of 29 individuals. BMC Musculoskelet Disord 2010;11:41.

59. Stevens M, Tan CW. Effectiveness of the Alfredson protocol compared with a lower repetition-volume protocol for midportion Achilles tendinopathy: a randomized controlled trial. J Orthop Sports Phys Ther 2014;44:59–67.

60. Silbernagel KG, Thomeé R, Thomeé P, et al. Eccentric overload training for patients with chronic Achilles tendon pain—a randomised controlled study with reliability testing of the evaluation methods. Scand J Med Sci Sports 2001;11: 197–206.

61. Malliaras P, Barton CJ, Reeves ND, et al. Achilles and patellar tendinopathy loading programmes: a systematic review comparing clinical outcomes and identifying potential mechanisms for effectiveness. Sports Med 2013;43:267–86.

62. Lian OB, Engebretsen L, Bahr R. Prevalence of jumper's knee among elite athletes from different sports: a cross-sectional study. Am J Sports Med 2005;33: 561–7.

63. Scott A, Ashe MC. Common tendinopathies in the upper and lower extremities. Curr Sports Med Rep 2006;5:233–41.

64. Zwerver J, Bredeweg SW, van den Akker-Scheek I. Prevalence of jumper's knee among nonelite athletes from different sports: a cross-sectional survey. Am J Sports Med 2011;39:1984–8.

65. Kongsgaard M, Qvortrup K, Larsen J, et al. Fibril morphology and tendon mechanical properties in patellar tendinopathy: effects of heavy slow resistance training. Am J Sports Med 2010;38:749–56.

Index

Note: Page numbers of article titles are in **boldface** type.

Clin Sports Med 34 (2015) 375–380
http://dx.doi.org/10.1016/S0278-5919(15)00011-3
0278-5919/15/$ – see front matter © 2015 Elsevier Inc. All rights reserved.

sportsmed.theclinics.com

Moving?

Make sure your subscription moves with you!

To notify us of your new address, find your **Clinics Account Number** (located on your mailing label above your name), and contact customer service at:

Email: journalscustomerservice-usa@elsevier.com

800-654-2452 (subscribers in the U.S. & Canada)
314-447-8871 (subscribers outside of the U.S. & Canada)

Fax number: 314-447-8029

Elsevier Health Sciences Division
Subscription Customer Service
3251 Riverport Lane
Maryland Heights, MO 63043

*To ensure uninterrupted delivery of your subscription, please notify us at least 4 weeks in advance of move.

Printed and bound by CPI Group (UK) Ltd, Croydon, CR0 4YY

03/10/2024

01040489-0020